INTIMATE ADVERSARIES

Cultural Conflict Between Doctors and Women Patients

Alexandra Dundas Todd

upp

UNIVERSITY OF PENNSYLVANIA PRESS

Philadelphia

Library of Congress Cataloging-in-Publication Data

Todd, Alexandra Dundas.
  Intimate adversaries.

  Bibliography: p.
  Includes index.
  1. Physician and patient.   2. Women patients—Psychol-
ogy.   3. Interpersonal conflict.   I. Title.
R727.3.T63   1989   610.69'6   88-27957
ISBN 0-8122-8152-7
ISBN 0-8122-1277-0 (pbk.)

Designed by Adrianne Onderdonk Dudden

2nd printing, 1990

0126114

Intimate Adversaries

For Drew

Contents

Acknowledgments

"The loneliness of the long-distance runner" is simultaneously the most appropriate and inappropriate metaphor for the writing of this book. On one hand, it brings to mind long hours spent alone, some glorious, some excruciating, moving toward a goal at times elusive, at times imminent. On the other hand, this book, like most books, is a social product, the result of a multitude of contributions from friends and colleagues.

I am enormously grateful to the following people for the interest they brought to this project. Will Wright and Sue Fisher offered their help and suggestions from the beginning to the end of the study. Rosemary Taylor and Nicole Rafter encouraged me to turn the research into a book, and I have benefited from their critical interest. Joined more recently but with equal intensity by Stephen Fox, these friends read drafts and provided a model for how exciting intellectual exchange can be.

Others contributed by reading individual chapters, offering editorial suggestions, or stimulating conversation. I would like to thank Rae Lesser Blumberg, Kate Ermenc, Joseph Gusfield, Robert Hahn, Evelyn Fox Keller, Jane Leserman, Bud Mehan, Joseph Rouse, Catherine Ryan, Wendy Sanford, Marlie Wasserman, and Irving Zola. I also want to thank all of the people—medical staff and women patients—who agreed to participate in this study; Suffolk University reference librarians Kathy Maio and Joe Middleton; secretarial staff Cindy Morley, Annalisa Kebadjian, and Frank Pellegrino; and Patricia Smith, editor at the University of Pennsylvania Press, who has made the publishing process smooth and steady.

My son, Drew Todd, in his usual wonderful way, offered his enthusiasm for and pride in my career, leading me to believe that behind every happy, successful, single parent stands a supportive child.

Introduction

Time magazine, in the late 1960s, boldly asked, "Is God Dead?" This question sent shock waves through homes and offices, creating controversy at every level of American life. The high priests of religion were said to be losing ground. Today, in the 1980s, when "post-industrial prophets" (Kuhns 1971) have asserted that science is the guiding light for modern society, a similar question might be asked: "Is science dead?" The answer to these queries is both yes and no. Religion is still very much with us, and a scientific view provides much of our conceptual appreciation of the world. But in recent years skepticism about science has grown, particularly with regard to medical science. Doctors, the most highly visible applied scientists, experience this skepticism perhaps most acutely. Scandals abound in research, and medical mistakes regularly make front-page copy. We all have our own personal stories of medical heresy. This represents a dramatic shift.

For much of this century, Americans have placed their faith in doctors and in the prevailing medical system. Such post World War II breakthroughs as the development of antibiotics and Jonas Salk's heralded polio vaccine provided credibility for modern medicine and increased public confidence. It was believed that cures were available for most ills and, if not, their discovery was just around the corner. In only a matter of time human disease would be completely eradicated through scientific research and expert medical care.[1]

Growing up in the 1950s, I found these views reflected in my family. The family doctor was called when needed and listened to with great respect. The mention of the men who had performed assorted family surgeries brought a near reverential hush to the conversation (malpractice cases were rare).[2] In sum, trust in doctors as the knowers and interpreters of scientific medical truth was intact.

Since the late 1960s, this trust has eroded. Skepticism toward authority in general has increased, and medicine is no exception. There is an increasing awareness on the part of the general public that a more selective eye needs to examine how doctors care for patients; and the regard for scientific medicine, which knew no bounds, has shown some limits. Doctors, who were thought to know all, are being questioned. The surgeries and drug therapies that used to be viewed as heroic and lifesaving increasingly are viewed with suspicion, needing the reinforcement of second opinions. Women, the major consumers of health care in this country, have been in the vanguard of these criticisms, which reflect such complaints as the overprescription of drugs, unnecessary surgeries, and biased medical attitudes toward women. Blind trust in modern medicine has waned. This is not to imply that modern medicine makes no contribution to health and life or that the majority of Americans criticize their medical care. The cry of dissent is a small voice slowly growing louder, not a full roar. But there have been few large-scale miracles and many failures for doctors in recent years. The public's expectations are high, often fueled by media extravaganzas on high-tech discoveries, and they are all too often dashed by daily realities. For example, although hearts can be surgically replaced, cures for most chronic illnesses remain elusive. Short of a cure for the common cold, at the very least, or, more important, for AIDS or cancer, medicine's magic is in trouble.

This movement in popular opinion from total trust to growing skepticism is mirrored in academic research. Talcott Parsons in the early 1950s wrote of the benevolent, nonmercenary expertise of modern medicine. More recent research has exposed the medical system to be flawed from its institutional and economic organization to the way doctors and patients communicate. The pedestal on which modern, scientific medicine stood is crumbling, being retitled the "clay pedestal" (Preston 1981). At the heart of these problems lies the doctor-patient relationship—the topic of this book.

Recent books on medical relationships, such as Paul Starr's (1982) historical analysis of current changes in the medical system and David Hilfiker's (1985) moving portrayal of doctors' difficulties in delivering health care, focus on the role and problems of doctors in our medical system. In this book I also look at medical relationships, but the focus changes. My primary interest is the patient—particularly when the patient is a woman.

Health care is a series of relationships among people, technologies, historical influences, and societal trends. In this book data are brought to bear on the doctor-patient relationship and what patients report they need and receive from their medical care. Whether a brief encounter between strangers in a clinic or hospital emergency room, rotational visits with interns and residents in a teaching hospital, annual checkups with the family physician in private practice, or the more customer-oriented treatment given in the newer corporate hospital, health care at its core is a face-to-face, person-to-person interaction.

This interaction takes place among individuals, but it would be misleading to reduce their meetings to the people directly involved. Rather, they are tied to complex attitudes and assumptions in the society in which they take place. Larger questions of organizational and structural influences on medical care and the more abstract, difficult-to-grasp world views that are embedded in cultural assumptions about the body, health, and social life are related to the ways people interact with each other in medical settings. The organization of American medicine is reflected in medical encounters, which, in turn, can reinforce and influence broader societal attitudes and structures. My interest here is to explore these dynamics. To study the problems between doctors and patients without considering the larger social contexts is to risk an overly simplistic analysis of a medical system composed of "bad" doctors and "complaining" patients.

It has long been the tradition in sociology to study either broad, large-scale considerations *or* social detail. Rarely are the two studied in tandem or connected in any meaningful way. Yet in social life the structure of society and culture is inextricably connected to daily experience. This book examines these connections and the impact they have on our understanding of the way health care is delivered in the United States.

My purpose here, then, is twofold. The doctor-patient relationship provides the substantive focus of the book. There is also a methodological interest in broadening the scope of sociological investigation to include different levels of analysis. Diverse literatures and approaches are brought to bear on the topic to enrich both understanding of the doctor-patient relationship and methods of sociological inquiry.

When the patient is a woman, additional areas for discussion arise. All of the dissatisfactions and problems discussed in the general doctor-patient relationship (Chapter 1) become exacerbated in the doctor–female patient relationship (Chapter 2).[3] Feminist scholars have revived scholarship on this topic during the last fifteen years, and more recently a growing literature is exploring the process of communication and/or interaction between women and their doctors.

Whether discussing the doctor-patient or doctor–female patient relationship, the epistemological underpinnings stemming from the medical model assume an interventionary treatment of biological disease, necessitating that people, men and women, enter the sick role for a cure. The prevailing view of patients is that they are, in varying degrees, ill. To the extent that they are sick, they have lost some control over their lives and normal routine activities, and this control is in part transferred to the doctor. Controversy exists over just how much control the medical profession should have over sick patients and how much control patients should retain over their treatment and thus their lives. This controversy centers around the situation of an ill person who needs treatment to be able to return to the patterns of normal life. It is this acute notion of disease that doctors are best equipped to handle. Women's health care, however, has a unique dimension. Reproductive processes are not illnesses, but rather a part of women's daily social lives. Healthy women go to the doctor for contraception and are treated individually as patients in a disease framework for matters that are biological, social, and interactive and that do not necessitate the shifts in routine life required by the sick role. Women seeking reproductive services are not, for the most part, ill. Yet today women enter the patient role and the care of a surgeon (obstetrician-gynecologist) to obtain these services. There is a difference in perspective here.

Neither doctors nor women patients tend to focus on or even be aware of this disjuncture between prevailing medical understandings and women's reproductive experiences. Rather, these are background noises so familiar to us that in everyday life they go unnoticed. My purpose in making noticeable the unnoticeable is to open yet another avenue to better understanding of medical relationships and women's lives.

My two-and-one-half-year study of audiotaped and observed communications between gynecologists and women patients in a private practitioner's office and a community clinic (Chapters 3 and 4) provides a close-up view of what takes place in medical interactions centered on reproductive care, primarily contraception. Contraception provides a rich area for investigation. First, it is a breach in the disease-focused medical model—contraceptive needs do not usually raise questions of illness. This breach clarifies the model under investigation. The imperfect fit between contraception and medical assumptions highlights rough edges. Second, women go to their doctors today in the wake of the women's movement and the so-called sexual revolution to seek help with their sexuality as well as with the explosive decisions of whether or not to have babies. Women run up against a medical system that is not organized around these questions but instead focuses on the technical and the diseased to the exclusion of the social context and on the individual to the exclusion of the familial or interactive. Although it can be argued that this latter approach is limited for all health care, involving diseases or nondiseases, it is certainly inappropriate for the well care needed for reproductive decision making. Contraception, then, illuminates problems in the doctor-patient relationship in general and the doctor–female patient relationship in particular.

To explore the dynamics of medical relationships, sociolinguistic methods are used to study the ways doctors and women communicate, or rather, all too often, miscommunicate. The medical interactions take varying forms, exposing details often missed in discussions of the medical system. For example, the negotiation between doctors and patients of topics to be discussed leads to interesting observations. Doctors concentrate on a biomedical approach to the body or organ. For patients, biological concerns are embedded in broader contextual experiences, especially when reproductive decisions are being made. This subtle clash in perspectives goes largely unexamined by participants or researchers. People, even when actively critical of their care, tend to focus on the insensitivity or coldness of doctors, the large amounts of money spent for short amounts of time, and so forth. Less often addressed is the subtler question of which topics are allowed and which are not allowed in medical conversations. It is observations such as these that move the analysis toward a consideration of the cultural assumptions that influence the practice of medicine (Chapter 5).

Explanations for the problems faced in our health care system range from criticisms of the profit and power motives that surround the medical-industrial establishment to the sexism that exists within patriarchal society and the practice of medicine. These explanations are crucial but not enough. In this book the analysis moves from detailed discussion of doctors and women patients talking about reproductive health to a broader discussion of medical organization and attitudes toward women. This is still not enough. I continue to an additional explanation of the problems that plague modern medicine. Both the scientific world view (which separates the mechanical body from the conscious mind) in modern Western societies and practical scientific considerations have greatly influenced contemporary medicine. It is this influence that most interests me. Although I touch on the importance of capitalism and discuss patriarchal attitudes, these areas have already been widely addressed. It is the relationship of a scientific world view to modern medicine and to women that is the core of this book. Writers in political economy and feminist theory have contributed in-depth analyses of society and medicine. Less has been said on the relationship among the epistemological roots of science, the development of the medical model, and the treatment of women patients. Connections are thus made here among the way people talk to each other, the model of modern American medicine, and some of the concepts about human beings and bodies which came out of the scientific revolution (starting in the West roughly in the sixteenth and seventeenth centuries). By combining detailed interactional data with an analysis of broader cultural assumptions about science and women, I provide the reader with an expanded view of the complexities of our medical system—complexities that shape and are shaped by the doctor-patient relationship.

This book is addressed to people who are or may become patients as well as to policy makers and sociologists. It is also addressed to doctors, although as a group they have been the least likely to show interest. One may give a talk on the doctor-patient relationship to a conservative women's luncheon, an academic conference, a feminist patient-centered medical collective, a business meeting, or a group of nonphysician medical professionals and workers, and the audience's reaction is largely the same. People can hardly contain their need to express their own rage at what they have experienced personally or seen in medical care. The most conservative sociologists, who would rebel against a radical critique of society, will rail against their treatment at the hands of doctors. The only group in society that refutes such talk is doctors themselves. Their first response, all too often, is that the research findings or criticisms (and they are overwhelmingly critical) are the exaggerated tales of complaining, neurotic women or radical, ivory tower academics, or that these are all exceptions to a normally unproblematic relationship in a well-functioning system. Thus doctors who are the group that most needs to hear what patients and critics are saying, are the least likely group to be listening. All of us, all too often, misunderstand each other. The doctor-patient relationship, however, carries a special impetus to avoid such misunderstandings—it can mean the difference, for the doctor, in job satisfaction or dissatisfaction, a malpractice suit or a referring patient, anguish or peace of mind; and for the patient the stakes are even higher. It can contribute to control or lack of control over reproductive processes, it can improve or decrease health; it can mean life or death. It is in our interests to understand better this relationship in all its complexities from the interactional, discursive level to structural, cultural influences. A close examination of medical relationships can have important consequences for us all.

NOTES

1. Ironically, although modern medicine and society historically have fallen short of such optimistic goals, and amid growing public pessimism, news headlines today from time to time trumpet the arrival of the new cure for all disease—gene transfer and therapy. Once past the headline, of course, we learn that this research

is still in its early stages and carries possibilities for as much disaster as delight (For example, "A World Without Disease," *Boston Globe*, January 27, 1985).

2. We tend to think medical malpractice suits are a new phenomenon, and to a great extent in regard to large awards this is true. Starr (1982) reminds us, however, that in the second half of the nineteenth century and the early years of this century, malpractice was a medical concern. Medical societies attracted doctors into their ranks by providing defense funds and services, winning the majority of cases for their members.

3. I have chosen not to address cases in which the doctor is a woman. The small amounts of data available are contradictory. This issue will become increasingly researchable as larger numbers of women medical students enter the work force. It will be some time before we know to what extent and in what quantity women physicians reach positions of decision making and administrative power. And once they are in these positions, only time will tell to what extent women do make or are allowed to make a difference.

1 | *The Heart of Medicine*

Sir Patrick: You mean to tell me you dont remember the woman with the tuberculous ulcer on her arm?

Ridgeon (enlightened): Oh, your washerwoman's daughter. Was her name Jane Marsh? I forgot.

Sir Patrick: Perhaps youve forgotten also that you undertook to cure her with Koch's tuberculin.

Ridgeon: And instead of curing her, it rotted her arm right off. Yes, I remember. Poor Jane! However, she makes a good living out of that arm now by shewing it at medical lectures.

Conversation between two doctors in *The Doctor's Dilemma* by George Bernard Shaw, 1909

We are told that our health care system is in trouble. A rapidly growing literature on the doctor-patient relationship has been receiving increasing public and professional attention, reinforcing this view. Scholarship on the medical system, including studies of actual communication between provider and patient, uncovers systematic dissatisfaction with the medical relationship and with health care in general. Modern medicine shines in many areas of acute care, yet patients complain of impersonal, overly technical treatment by uncaring doctors. Doctors report that patients behave immaturely and ignore recommendations. Not all encounters are problematic, but, as will be discussed, regardless of individual attributes, the doctor-patient relationship, the heart of medicine, occurs in a strained context. It involves a network of relationships that reach inside and outside of daily interactions, stretching out to cultural and societal assumptions and back to conversations centered on specific topics related to health. In this chapter external influences on medical encounters will be examined briefly. Then dynamics between doctors and patients within medical settings will be reviewed.

OUTSIDE LOOKING IN

The very organization of American health care contributes to the problems currently voiced about the doctor-patient relationship. The political economy of a health care system run for profit, a limited medical model and definition of health, and a medical education that reinforces this model have all been brought into the spotlight for critical examination. In this section these external forces will be explored for their relationship to doctors and patients.

The Political Economy of Health Care

The economics of American medicine, all too often emphasizing profits rather than health, have long been seen as an integral influence on the quality, or lack thereof, of health care. George Bernard Shaw's skepticism when discussing turn-of-the-century British medicine is timely for the present American system:

> It is not the fault of our doctors that the medical service of the community, as at present provided for, is a murderous absurdity. That any sane nation, having observed that you could provide for the supply of bread by giving bakers a pecuniary interest in baking for you, should go on to give a surgeon a pecuniary interest in cutting off your leg, is enough to make one despair of political humanity. But that is precisely what we have done. And the more appalling the mutilation, the more the mutilator is paid. He who corrects the ingrowing toenail receives a few shillings: he who cuts your inside out receives hundreds of guineas, except when he does it to a poor person for practice. . . . I cannot knock my shins severely without forcing on some surgeon the difficult question, "Could I not make a better use of a pocketful of guineas than this man is making of his leg?" (Shaw 1909:3)

Shaw's remarks were aimed at early twentieth-century England, but he would most likely turn an equally scathing eye on American medicine today.

Medical critics argue that the structure of medical care mirrors the structure of American society—it is hierarchical in the organization of its professional workers and in its delivery of health care; it is based on profit and functions through inequality. In fact, the seeking of profit runs like a steady stream through American medical care, as it does through the rest of the society. The power base of the medical establishment is a well-protected fortress, with profits providing the carefully guarded crown jewels. The business enterprises that market health-related goods and services—the pharmaceutical companies, health insurance and medical supply industries, proprietary hospitals and nursing homes, and to a large extent the practice of medicine itself with doctors among the highest paid professionals in the country—are tremendously profitable. The strength of this orientation toward profit is evident in a simple fact: with the exception of South Africa, the United States is the only industrialized country to have no form of nationalized health care.

Many in the population in need of our expensive health services are underserved or not served at all. We have a two-class medical system offering the best and the worst. Thus the delivery of health care varies widely. For some, even basic care is nonexistent. For others, with financial means, particularly those in need of high-tech solutions for complicated but solvable problems, it is lifesaving. The majority, who fall in between these two extremes, hold complex attitudes toward the quality of care received and the price paid. As medicine increasingly is taken over by large corporate, for-profit interests, these problems are expected to increase dramatically (see Chapter 6).

The political and economic history of our health care delivery system is, however, more complex than a critique of profit mongering (see Stevens 1971, Starr 1982). For example, the government intervened to improve health care facilities with the Hill-Burton Act in the 1940s and medical access by creating Medicare and Medicaid in the 1960s, as well as encouraging community efforts to bring care to the people. These efforts improved availability for some but fell short of the goal; equity in health care remains elusive.[1] Costs continue to rise alarmingly, making progressive change more difficult. For various reasons insurance companies, business, and government are calling for increased regulation of the health care system. Physicians, beleaguered from all sides, are often at the center of calls for reform because they are seen as pivotal in the control of rising costs. These calls can place them in the position of pitting costs against patients' needs. At the same time legal interventions (especially the rise in malpractice cases) pressure doctors to practice more defensively, and defensive practices can further increase their distance from patients (Taylor 1984).

In the late 1980s we see an ironic shift in medical perspective that contributes further to this distance. The medical profession, which for most of this century has called for trust from the public and has claimed objective superiority based on scientific expertise over all alternative medicines, is now, in the wake of malpractice, claiming that medicine is an "inexact science." "The public's expectations are too high." The profession finds itself caught in a contradiction. On one hand it wants to hold onto the scientific optimism, the status, and the societal and economic privilege garnered since World War II, and on the other hand it denies responsibility for the powers on which these privileges are based. The public, becoming confused about what to expect, usually expects too much based on past promises and ends up angry when outcomes fall short. An imbalance in expectations exists between doctors and patients before they even meet. This struggle is intricately tied to the political and economic trends in society and medicine. Profits, status, hierarchy, and the need for control are incompatible with egalitarian medical relationships (for a more detailed discussion of these topics see Doyal 1979, Ehrenreich 1978, Ehrenreich and Ehrenreich 1971, Navarro 1976, 1986, Waitzkin 1983).

The economic system is one influence on the shape of the health care delivery system and the doctor-patient relationship. Another influence, subtler but equally important, resides at the level of culture and involves ways of knowing, ways of seeing that are embodied in the often elusive qualities of the *model* of medicine used in contemporary Western societies. An examination of this model reveals the basic assumptions upon which the modern practice of medicine depends.

The Medical Model

The biomedical model is pervasive in our society—so pervasive that it goes unnoticed. One of the interests of social critics is to change the assumed to the examined, and Siegler and Osmond (1974) begin this revelation by delineating two central aspects of modern Western medicine. The first is the concept of the "Aesculapian authority" of the doctor, and the second is the notion of the "sick role" of the patient—a concept they borrow from Parsons (1951).

In Greek mythology Aesculapius was the first physician, the overseer of Greek health, and was elevated to the status of the gods. Aesculapian authority is a right to power based on superior knowledge, moral authority, and charismatic authority. In Western medicine the doctor has traditionally been awarded a lofty position based on superior knowledge, technical skill, and a scientific halo to bolster charismatic qualities.

Medical authority comes, then, not from brute force over people's lives but from a subtler control based on a belief system that assumes doctors' superiority (see Paul Starr's discussion of cultural authority 1982: 13–15). The patient plays a very important part in the maintenance of this idealized relationship, for it is the patient who in this century has internalized trust for the doctor's expertise. An ideology of the need for dependence on experts has been in evidence for most of the century. The roles doctors and patients play are just one example of this trend whereby the ill person enters the sick role for medical treatment. The patient enters a passive, childlike role in need of care by the wiser, more knowledgeable, expert doctor (see Parsons 1951, Siegler and Osmond 1974).

Elliot Mishler (1981) further delineates the "silent assumptions" of the medical model by pointing out that disease is theoretically based on specific etiology and represents a deviation from the norm. In our model of medicine the biological fact is diagnosed and cured under the rubric of an objectively neutral scientific model. The body or organ separated from the mind is considered the seat of disease and is the locus of medical attention. The person-host to the disease is passive, temporarily on hold until the malfunctioning part is fixed: "Thus the biomedical model embraces both reductionism, the philosophic view that complex phenomena are ultimately derived from a single primary principle, and mind-body dualism, the doctrine that separates the mental from the somatic" (Engel 1977 : 130).

The assumptions of this model influence how medical training educates doctors to think about health, illness, and patients. Many of the dissatisfactions present in today's doctor-patient relationship can be traced back to these underlying assumptions. George Engel points out that as this approach to disease intersects with a profit orientation, the doctor-patient relationship suffers: "The power of vested interests, social, political, and economic, are formidable deterrents to any effective assault on biomedical dogmatism. . . . The enormous existing and planned investment in diagnostic and therapeutic technology alone strongly favors approaches to clinical study and care of patients that emphasize the impersonal and the mechanical" (1977:135). As we shall see in later chapters, rapport between participants and improved health are at risk in such narrow understandings.

Medical Education

Along with biotechnical training, doctors receive a subtler lesson in dominance from their medical education, encouraging a superior approach to the patients' views. Doctors' and patients' behaviors are separated into basically two different categories—expert (doctor) and layperson (patient). Patients are defined as incapable of understanding their bodies. Such a definition provides little grounds for medical respect. My observations of two medical schools' practicum training programs show one aspect of the subtle socialization medical students experience to become doctors. These medical students' introductions to clinical care took place in veterans' hospitals. The students, predominantly white, middle and upper class, young, and healthy, treated patients who tended to be multiracial, lower-middle, working, and lower class, elderly, chronically ill, and resentful at being used as teaching material. The rationale that such a patient population provided comprehensive teaching experience may be true. There was, however, an additional lesson learned: patients are different, patients are difficult, and patients are inferior.[2]

When participating in a medical school class on sexuality to help orient future doctors to more effective ways of dealing with people's problems, I observed another medical lesson. The course was introduced with some basic "porn flicks" (as they were called) to familiarize students with all the possible "aberrations" in sexual behavior. These were shown with the air of a carnival, with popcorn served and jokes throughout. The other four sessions concentrated on technical aspects of sexual biology. Such information as changes in millimeters of the vagina before and after female orgasm was discussed at length in a slide presentation. It seems unlikely that this is a topic much raised by patients when consulting doctors about their sexuality. Neither the high splash of the sex films nor the technical lectures taught doctors what they would need to answer the more likely complaints of sexual insecurity or impotence. In my research it was exactly these questions that patients all too frequently tacked embarrassedly onto the end of a medical consultation and which were dismissed by equally embarrassed physicians on their way out the door.

Furthermore, while experimental programs are beginning, there is little incentive for medical students to explore social-psychological topics in more depth. Medical students are so inundated with scientific and technical information that there is some question whether they will be able to add yet new areas even when schools do offer them. Although Derek Bok, President of Harvard University, calls for a change in perspective in medical education, improved technical approaches still rank highest as the path to success. A recent poll of Harvard Medical School faculty and students disclosed that the four skills seen as most in need of bolstering reinforce a dehumanizing and technological framework around medical care. None of them addresses the need for social and interpersonal skills.[3]

External influences such as political and economic arrangements, the biomedical model, and medical education affect the doctor-patient relationship. But what actually happens in face-to-face encounters between doctors and patients? What are the internal structures of this relationship and what do they mean for health? To reveal a better understanding of exactly what goes on and what goes wrong in this relationship, a few researchers have focused on patients' perceptions and the structure of interactions between physicians and the people who go to them for health care.

MOVING INWARD

Mallory walked in and sat down on the empty chair next to the bed, throwing his right arm over the chair back as if he had all day to chat. He tried to give the impression that he was at leisure to talk about anything and everything. At the same time he tried to keep his visits to three minutes per patient.

"Well, Mrs. Rosen, how are you doing today?" he said.

"I'm scared." She had a pale, narrow face and a cloud of black hair. She flipped through the pages of the magazine and put it down. "Wait, I have a list of questions for you."

"Terrific." Inwardly, Mallory cursed. These written lists of questions took too much time. . . . This habit of writing down questions had been diagnosed as a secondary disease in the latest *New England Journal of Medicine:* "La Maladie du Petits Papiers."

Susan Cheever, Doctors and Women, 1987

Much has been said on the structure of medical care—the system and how it meshes with, reflects, and reinforces the larger society. Not much is said about what actually happens within the practice(s) of medicine, but examination of one-on-one interactions between people provides a fluid rather than a static understanding of society and daily life. In other words, there is a negotiation process that is always at work in the creation and maintenance of social values and institutions. As Paula Treichler and her colleagues so aptly state,

> Though we acknowledge that such "preconditions" as status, gender, and race influence participants' attitudes and expectations, we suggest that it is also important to examine the *interactive behavior* of the participant. Power as a dynamic concept emerges within patterns of communication over time and space, and cannot be located as a property of the individual. Rather, power becomes the negotiated product of a mutually constituted and mutually administered interaction system. From this standpoint, any assessment of power must take the details of interaction . . . into account. (1984:63–64)

Power and face-to-face interaction are seen as intricately entwined. In this spirit Chapters 3, 4, and 5 draw out the connections between what goes on in the everyday world of experience and elements of the larger society. At this point, however, it is important to review what is known about the inside workings of the doctor-patient relationship and what transpires in the everyday world of health care.

Studies reveal that the average doctor visit lasts 15.4 minutes, with 47 percent lasting 10 minutes or less and 74 percent lasting 15 minutes or less. Only 6 percent last more than 30 minutes. This does not allow much time to deliver a diagnosis, prognosis, and treatment, not to mention education and advice, or to elicit people's views (Hingson et al. 1981). Increasingly, technology is called upon for assistance if for no other reason (and there are other reasons) than to save valuable time. The very way the system is organized limits the possibility of interpersonal skills and attention to the psychosocial dynamics of illness. Korsch et al. (1968) found that time was not as important as it often is supposed for improving the doctor-patient relationship (that is, if the doctor did not have good communication skills; tacking more time on the length of the interview was not a solution), but the lack of time does hinder the development of interactional competence on the parts of both doctors and patients. Using good communication skills, however, does *not* take more office time according to Korsch. In fact, it seems logical that these skills could shorten time needed to elicit and impart information.

Many doctors are frustrated, however, by time shortages—time shortages that begin in the hectic years of medical school, when large doses of information are administered at breakneck speed. This pace does not slow down as the student progresses to thirty-six-hour rotations in big city public hospital emergency rooms during internship and residency. The message is that time is in short supply, it can mean life, it can mean death, it can mean bureaucratic efficiency, and it always means money.

An important factor in the doctor-patient relationship is that patients are usually sick and doctors are usually healthy. Illness is always anxiety-provoking and emotionally difficult. The patient is a stranger in a strange land, where only a small minority understand the gadgets, procedures, and options; for doctors the territory is familiar. If time constraints and economic considerations are added, the result is a relationship that begins in struggle.

Doctor-Patient Communication

In social science literature the doctor-patient relationship is traditionally described as asymmetrical, with dominating doctors and passive patients participating in a "ceremony" of sickness (see Freidson 1970, Parsons 1951, Strong 1979, Waitzkin and Waterman 1974, Zola 1972). A close scrutiny of this relationship and medical discourse has revealed how doctor-patient communication maintains the inequality of the relationship (Fisher and Todd 1983, Strong 1979). Not only have doctors traditionally regulated who enters the medical system and who does not, they continue to control the transmission of information once the patient is in the system. If the patient belongs to a racial minority, this control intensifies. As Roger Shuy, one of the few researchers to address the question of race in medical discourse, concludes in a recent discussion of black patients, "Consciously or unconsciously, dialect speakers tend to get worse treatment, wait longer for service, are considered ignorant, and are told what to do rather than asked what they would like to do" (1983:192). Thus while reviewing the literature on doctor-patient communication, it is important to note that race and class differences affect this relationship.

Byrne and Long (1976), in 2,500 doctor-patient interviews in England, found that "doctor-centered," "information-gathering" conversations were the most prevalent modes of talk. Biomedical information was gathered with little listening or reflecting on the part of the doctors. Byrne and Long found hardly any allowance for patient-centered concerns to emerge once the initial complaint was stated. The minority of three doctors who used a patient-centered style spent time listening to the patient, reflecting on the talk, and allowing for silences so patients could insert topics of their own. Any teacher interested in student participation will verify that a classroom without pauses or silences is a classroom without spontaneous student contributions. The same seems to be true of the medical interview.

Shuy's (1974) research, based on transcribed doctor-patient interactions, also shows the interview to be dominated by the doctor's medical language and perspective. Patients intimidated by this talk tried to imitate it, failed, and returned to their own language. This failure for the patient has the possible outcome of leading to even vaguer, more flustered talk. Shuy found the interviews efficient and technically adequate but emotionally or empathetically lacking. Similarly, Korsch et al. (1968), studying a pediatric outpatient clinic, found few civilities. Discussions were dominated by technical information, with little emotion shown. The psychosocial aspects of patients' lives or illnesses were generally ignored, with the doctors asking questions and the patients providing answers. Candace West (1984) also discusses the doctor's role as questioner and the patient's role as answerer revealing the linguistic dominance of the doctor. In the data presented in Chapter 3, there is a basic irony—the patient comes to the doctor with questions about her health, but the doctor asks all the questions.

Patient-Doctor Dissatisfactions

The situation that emerges from these studies is a doctor-dominated, biomedical orientation in the provider-patient relationship. What about the patient? Although the research is by no means complete in these areas, what is available tells us that dissatisfaction does exist among patients. David Mechanic (1968) found that roughly one-third of the people interviewed in one community said they changed medical care because of dissatisfaction with their primary provider. Reasons most cited were mistaken diagnosis, unsuccessful treatment, and detachment or perceived lack of concern on the part of doctors for people's problems. Korsch's research teams (1968, 1972) show similar findings in studies of pediatric patients and their mothers in emergency rooms. Of the mothers who reported dissatisfaction, 70 percent cited doctors' disinterest in their concerns. In eight hundred emergency room examinations, half the mothers said they left not knowing what caused their child's illness, and close to one-fifth were not clear about what was currently wrong with their child. The researchers' analyses of these interactions verify the mothers' versions that the doctors did not impart this information. Furthermore, less than 6 percent of the doctors' talk was categorized as warm or friendly. All of this contributed to feelings of helplessness and anxiety on the part of the mothers. The result can be problems for the child's health. At home it is the mother who will be in charge of care, and her self-confidence and understanding of the illness rather than self-doubt is crucial.

People's confusion about medical care is prevalent in the above sample of studies. A thread that runs through these reports is a quality of demoralization. People expressed dissatisfaction when their own views were ignored, unsolicited, or both. Although a good doctor must be a good technician, patients' satisfaction is also dependent on their being able to tell doctors stories in their own words—their understanding of what is going on in their own or their children's lives. It is also dependent on the doctor's reciprocating with clear information on the prognosis (Stiles et al. 1979). But Stone (1979) asserts that doctors do this poorly if at all. Either they lapse into medical jargon that may seem normal to them but is foreign to the patient or they take on a patronizing, simplistic style that insults the patient. Each route leaves much to be desired for medical communication and contributes to people's feelings of powerlessness.

Similar confusion seems to surround the content of the information that is given to patients. On one hand, doctors, to protect themselves from accusations of uninformed consent or malpractice, tell it all, often coldly, emphasizing the worst. On the other hand, there is the mum effect—doctors give little information, deciding the patient would not understand anyway or to avoid giving bad news (Rodin 1982).

> When a doctor perceives the patient as rather poorly informed, he considers the tremendous difficulties of translating his knowledge into language the patient can understand, along with dangers of frightening the patient; the patient, in turn, reacts fully to this limited information, either asking uninspired questions or refraining from questioning the doctor at all, thus reinforcing the doctor's view that the patient is ill-equipped to comprehend his problem. Lacking guidance, the patient performs at a low level; hence, the doctor rates his capacities as even lower than they are. (Pratt et al., in Hingson et al. 1981:146)

In defense of doctors, it should be recognized that they, too, have dissatisfactions in their relationships with patients. Doctors suffer frustration with this same lack of success coupled with the public's high expectations. David Hilfiker writes, "As practicing primary-care physicians, then, we work in an impossible situation. Each of the myriad decisions to be made every day has the potential for drastic consequences if it is not determined properly. . . . Any patient encounter can dump me back into the situation of having caused more harm than good, yet my role is to be a healer" (1984:121–22).

The medical profession's encouragement of the public's blind faith in doctors may have paid off in some respects, but such trust in the face of so many medical unknowns can prove difficult for doctors in everyday practice. A passage between a doctor and the American wife of a terminal leukemia patient in Harriet Doerr's novel *Stones for Ibarra* displays the difficulties that high expectations create for doctor-patient communication:

> When, at seven o'clock that morning, Dr. Vasquez had been called to the Evertons' bedroom, he took Richard's temperature and gave him an injection. The intern surveyed his patient from the foot of the bed. Sara stood there, too, expecting signs of immediate improvement. Richard was thin, having lived on broth and juice for three days. Now Sara waited for him to say "Please bring me toast and a boiled egg." Or, "I need graph paper and my slide rule."
>
> Dr. Vasquez examined the quiet profile of his patient's wife. When at last she looked in his direction, the set of her mouth and the absence of tears in her intent wide eyes confirmed his suspicion. The sick man's wife believed doctors had supernatural powers. She believed this of the American specialist and of Dr. Vasquez himself.
>
> He started to say, "I must make clear to you the serious nature of your husband's illness," but instead merely presented a report [on community activities].

Given such frustrations, burdens of time pressures, patients who expect too much, the risk of medical error (see Bosk 1979), and an inadequate education in the psychosocial realm of illness, it is no wonder that occupational stress for doctors is high. Doctors are more likely than the rest of the population to suffer high suicide rates, heart disease, alcoholism, and drug abuse. Cartwright (1967) correlates doctors' high levels of stress with difficulty in sitting still or slowing down long enough to hear patients through or really listen. Just as high anxiety may interfere with patients' really hearing what doctors have to say to them, high stress seems to have an impact on doctors' communication skills. Faced with such discomfort it becomes easier for both to fall back on prescribed roles—the doctor asks all the questions and the patient does all the answering.

The opposite extreme for doctors is often boredom. Medical practice is not all heart transplants and cutting-edge discoveries. Most of it entails repetitive routines—looking at the thirty-ninth infected ear in a week or treating the tenth case of vaginitis since lunch. The doctors I worked with talked of immense job satisfaction; but they also often found medical practice to be far more routine than they had imagined it would be when they started medical school.

In sum, doctor-patient communication is often miscommunication or noncommunication, with patients and doctors having just cause for complaint. Whether or not all of the above scenarios are played out between doctor and patient, this relationship is a setup. The potential for dissatisfaction is great. But what about health? People go to the doctor to improve their health. Does the communication gap make any difference to this goal? The findings to date, as well as my own research (Chapter 4), say that it does.

Communication and Health

Good communication skills between doctors and patients increase doctors' understanding of the problem and patients' understanding of the necessary treatment, and they influence recovery (Langer et al. 1975). Waitzkin and Stoeckle (1972) conclude that when doctors and patients are communicating well the results are (1) a better chance of good history taking, thus higher quality of medical care; (2) better medical records, particularly important in clinic or group practice; and (3) possible improvement in patients' psychological and physiological responses to medical treatment. Etiology and course of disease and even death have been connected to feelings of powerlessness and lack of control. More patient control equals improved health outcomes (Cousins 1979, Johnson 1975, Langer and Rodin 1976).

One ingredient in this greater control is information. Dorothy Wertz and colleagues (1984), in their study of 880 genetic counseling sessions lasting from forty to sixty minutes each, found a high rate of unawareness on the part of both counselor and client of the topic the other most wanted to discuss. In 47.5 percent of the sessions neither counselor (mostly doctors) nor client, after the session, reported correctly what the other wanted to discuss most; in 26.2 percent both parties had this knowledge; in 15.7 percent the counselor but not the client was aware; and in 10.6 percent the reverse was true. The researchers found that when all the participants were aware of what the other wanted to discuss, the sessions were the most effective. They conclude that if educationally oriented medicine is to improve, clients need education in understanding medical professionals, and, even more important, providers must hone their communication skills.

Information exchanges, however, raise long-standing debates among medical providers. How much information is appropriate? Howard Waitzkin's (1984) findings display some of the uncertainties. From 336 taped encounters in Massachusetts and California, doctors and patients were asked to rate patients' informational needs. In 65 percent of the interactions, patients' desires for information were underestimated by doctors (in 6 percent patients' desires were overestimated, and in 29 percent they were estimated correctly). The actual time doctors spent giving information to patients averaged about one minute in interactions lasting roughly twenty minutes. Doctors reported, however, that they spent more time giving information in these encounters than the data indicated. In other words, they overestimated this activity. A discrepancy exists between doctors' and patients' perceptions of the amount of information needed and given.

Adequate interactions, complicated as they may be, are crucial to the medical enterprise. Satisfactory exchanges of information have been significantly connected to improved health. Patients who properly understand what to expect cope better than do the uninformed. In a review of thirty-four controlled studies, Mumford, Schlesinger, and Glass (1982) found that when surgical or coronary patients were given information, support, or both to help them through medical procedures, they did better than patients who received routine care. Hospital stays were reduced, and recovery time can be decreased. Similar results have been shown in childbirth (Breen 1975, Levy and McGee 1975); difficult or painful physical examinations (Johnson and Leventhal 1974); and when the patient is a child (Wolfer and Vistainer 1975). Increased patient control and participation leads to better understanding of the problem and necessary treatment, often resulting in improved health care.

Compliance

A last point concerns the much highlighted, often elusive issue of patient compliance. Do patients, in this role socially defined as passive, do what they are told by their doctors? Many do, but many do not. Dunbar and Stunkard in their review of 165 studies on this subject found that between 20 and 82 percent of patients do not comply with their doctors' orders (in Mishler et al. 1981). Irving Zola (1980) points out that nearly 50 percent of patients do not comply with their medication treatment. This behavior and its great variability are influenced by type of illness, medical setting, and different types of patients, doctors, and treatment plans—much of which is beyond the control of any of the participants. There is also some evidence, however, that the inequalities and complexities in the doctor-patient relationship can have an impact. Ralph Hingson and his colleagues (1981) in their review of the literature on this subject maintain that patients are less likely to comply

(1) if they believe that they are not held in adequate esteem by their physicians,

(2) if their physicians actively seek information from them without providing feedback about either why that information is being gathered or on the patients' conditions,

(3) if tension emerges during a doctor-patient interaction and is not addressed or resolved, or

(4) if patients believe that their expectations are not being met or that their physicians are not behaving in a friendly manner. (1981:147)

Korsch and Negrete (1972), studying a working-class population, found that the higher number of supportive statements on the part of the doctor and the more sought-after information mothers received, the higher the likelihood of compliance. Charney et al. (1967) and Hulka et al. (1976) report similar findings in their studies of middle-class populations. Stone (1979) found that doctors' abilities to educate patients in necessary procedures, and the degree of empathy and caring expressed, decreased patients' anxiety and increased their cooperation. Waitzkin and Stoekle (1972) conclude in their research that the more one knows about his or her illness, the higher the rate of compliance. I would add that the more doctors encourage patients to contribute to the arranging of regimens, the more likely the recommendations will be followed. Patients, as will be discussed in later chapters, have relationships, work schedules, pressures, and so forth, which rarely emerge in medical conversations but which influence their handling of medical treatments. Only patients are in a position to insert this information into medical decision making. Thus, just as patients need information on their illnesses from doctors, doctors need information on the social parameters of treatment possibilities from patients. Put into equation form, this literature indicates that

Adequate exchange of information ⇄ understanding ⇄ better decision making ⇄ better health care delivery ⇄ "therapeutic alliance" (as Zola has so aptly reconceptualized compliance).

The startling lack of patient compliance has been a popular theme in medicine and the focus of much attention. What is interesting here is the framework in which this discussion takes place. Patients, from the medical perspective, are seen as the core of the problem—they are unsophisticated about medical treatments or they are too headstrong to follow instructions. The studies discussed here show that the doctor and the organization of medicine also contribute to this problem. Many of the skills needed to improve people's involvement are lacking in medical education and in the medical model under which health care is delivered. Doctors do not seem to comply with patients' needs any more than patients comply with doctors' treatments. Compliance is a negotiation between the participants. Perhaps patients' needs for respect and adequate exchange are not just demands for hand-holding, but a plea, even if unwittingly, for improved health care.

Just as doctors' compliance has not received much fanfare, neither has the question, Is it in patients' interests to comply? Franz Ingelfinger (1977) estimates that 80 percent of patients have problems that will either go away on their own or are untreatable; a little over 10 percent can be dramatically improved by modern medical techniques; and roughly 9 percent run the risk of being harmed. "So the balance of accounts ends up marginally on the positive side of zero" (in Preston 1981:115). Perhaps. There is, however, another way to interpret these figures. The 80 percent of patients who have self-contained diseases nonetheless often receive treatment—tests galore, drugs, even surgery. One 1983 presidential commission reports that 50 to 65 percent of antibiotics are perhaps unnecessarily prescribed or administered incorrectly, 20 percent of hospital days may be unwarranted, and billions of dollars are wasted each year in unnecessary tests, x-rays, and so forth (in Bok 1984:7). With such an overdose of treatments, a percentage of people will be harmed physically, emotionally, and financially. Because the system is set up for doctors to keep pushing the lure of a cure and for patients to keep coming back for more, shouldn't patients question medical advice?

CONCLUSION

At the heart of the medical profession, and crucial to its future, is the doctor-patient relationship. This relationship has the potential in part to shape and to be shaped by the directions medicine is taking (or being pushed into; see Chapter 6). It is important to understand that while we still, as a society, labor under an increasingly tarnished illusion of kindly medical relationships, in theory and in fact doctors and patients are locked in a semiadversarial relationship. Patients feel that doctors should make them better all of the time. Great expectations become easily thwarted. To doctors, patients often seem an erratic, unpredictable group who increasingly demand what doctors cannot give and often ignore what is prescribed. As Hilfiker so aptly describes, each patient presents the risk of medical mistake or misjudgment, leading to psychological stress and possibly high costs in money and reputation in the law courts.

The idealized version envisioned by earlier sociologists such as Talcott Parsons of the powerful, detached, godlike doctor who knows best, curing the passive patient, who turns all decision making over to higher authority, is outdated. Health seems to depend on a more equal relationship between two active participants involved in the often difficult task of problem solving and decision making. In our current organization of health care, however, is this possible? This question is of particular importance to women, for women are the major consumers of health care in America today. Women are also less likely than men to be seen as equal to the task of being treated equally.

NOTES

1. Presidents Dwight Eisenhower, John Kennedy, Lyndon Johnson, Richard Nixon, and Jimmy Carter in addresses to the public all asserted the need to make health care a right for all Americans (Ronald Reagan never shared this goal). De-

spite such interest, these promises have never been fulfilled. We still grapple with the following questions: Is health care a right or a privilege? Should health care within a free market system be treated as a commodity or a public good sequestered from market forces? (See Navarro 1986 and Waitzkin 1983 for detailed discussion of these questions. See Kleinman 1980 for a cross-cultural examination of health care systems.) It would be a mistake, however, to assume that efforts, though not achieving equity, have had no impact. Medicaid and Medicare have certainly made contributions to availability of health care for some. Starr in numerous lectures has pointed out the improvements in health the programs of the 1960s and 1970s delivered. Harrington (1984), though not satisfied with the poverty programs he helped create, nonetheless sees it as a mistake to think they did no good.

2. Daniel Segal's intriguing study, "Playing Doctor, Seriously: Graduation Follies at an American Medical School," depicts another aspect of the ingrained cultural values medical students receive by the end of four years of training: "The professional identity of physicians is constructed in terms of a conceptual principle that opposes 'the power to save lives' to 'the vulnerability of mere mortals,' and thus marks physicians as strong and patients as weak—the first as superiors, the second as inferiors. In sum, as they romped around the stage, both the disciples and their masters were playing doctor—seriously" (1984:395). Waitzkin and Waterman (1974) label this distance between doctors and patients the "competence gap." The groundwork for this gap begins in medical school training and contributes to doctors' control and patients' powerlessness.

3. Interestingly, Bok emphasizes the need for a more sensitive curriculum which addresses social and psychological aspects of health and medicine. Elsewhere in the report he lists the high ranking of these increased technical areas reported by doctors and students. He does this apparently unaware that a contradiction seems to exist between what he says he is advocating and what medical students and faculty are calling for.

2 | The Diseasing of Reproduction: When the Patient Is a Woman

Interviewer: How do you feel about doctors in general?

Respondent 1: I don't have a very high opinion of them in general right now. . . . Because they have so many patients, uh, they seem to be interested primarily in the money they're going to get out of you and their whole idea of medicine is come in, give you some chemicals.

Respondent 2: With the current bills that I have, I think they're all a bunch of rip-off artists.

Respondent 3: Doctors? As doctors, yuck, I don't like doctors. I think 99 percent of them are bullshit.

Respondent 4: I get a little uptight with [the] doctor because he sometimes gets into this pattern of forgetting the patient . . . he's only looking at the medical side of it.

In my data, from which the above excerpts are taken, the majority of the women I talked with (Chapters 3 and 4) had a low opinion of their medical care. Although they often cited positive experiences with individual doctors and staff, they had had enough negative interactions and results to foster feelings of discontent. Interestingly, the doctors in the two settings I studied were totally unaware of patient hostility. Because patients did not voice their dissatisfactions to doctors and because, understandably, doctors did not try to ferret out attitudes they did not know existed, these hostilities remained beneath the surface.

The sentiments of discontent that so color my data have been the subject of much debate in recent years. Doctors, in general, when faced with growing public criticism, voice their own complaints, often focusing on what they see as inadequacies in their patients. The women's health movement, an outgrowth of the feminist reawakening of the late 1960s, responded by focusing a penetrating and often critical eye on modern medicine's control of women's bodies. Feminist historians have, for example, criticized the social organization of reproduction and contraception. This has not been an easy task because most medical history has emphasized a male and medical bias, reinforcing present conventional understandings of the field. Thomas McKeown, a British medical historian, has pointed out that "historians of medicine, like historians of art have two main themes, the great men and the great movements" (1976:4). These themes have been developed at the expense of any social understanding of what health and disease have meant to people's, especially women's, lives or what McKeown refers to as public interest.

For example, from the medical perspective, J. Marion Sims, the nineteenth-century American physician hailed by medical historians as the "architect of the vagina," fits into the great men category. He is considered the father of gynecology, the inventor of gynecological surgery, and a savior of women and their health. This view of Sims went largely uncontested until the last decade, when other aspects of his medical practice were scrutinized. An alternative historical perspective reveals a man who practiced surgery on his slaves for four years (thirty operations on one slave alone) before taking his talents into "polite society." He literally built and rebuilt the vagina. We see a man driven by the desire for success, who found that diseases of the female reproductive organs could be a vehicle for fulfillment of this desire (see Barker-Benfield 1976). The real J. Marion Sims probably lies between these two portraits, but the first and more widely known picture is far too favorable.

In a similar vein, feminist scholars have contributed an alternative view of the historical rise of medical science, contributions not without controversies of their own. How we define historical events is debatable. Is history something that we study to understand past trends and influences on current events, or do we use our current understandings to interpret, and to some extent recreate, history? The answer is surely a dialogue between these possibilities. Differences in perspective by feminist scholars of the history of women's health care that emerged between the early 1970s and the 1980s illustrate this question.

In the late 1960s and early 1970s, when women again began articulating the limitations of women's roles in contemporary society, the emerging historical interpretation of women in the nineteenth century rendered them passive. Women were oppressed. They were seen as pawns in a man's game, be he father, husband, or doctor (Ehrenreich and English 1978). As the women's movement grew in this country, with a concomitant change in expected gender roles, and as women have become, in the 1980s, increasingly active in public and private spheres, the interpretation of this history has shifted slightly. To define women as passive recipients of society's and/or male dictates is seen as misrepresenting and underestimating women's strengths. The nineteenth-century woman, whether involved in struggle for social change or accepting of traditional values, is redefined as an active participant in her own life, even in her own oppression (albeit unwittingly). In other words, it is better to have been an active participant in the arrangement of one's life (regardless of how falsely conscious) than to be a passive being (see Leavitt 1984).

The important element here, regardless of which interpretation of women's lives takes precedence, is power—who has it, who does not. In the nineteenth century as in the twentieth, power has resided for the most part with some men rather than with women. Women, whether understood to be active or passive, have generally *responded to* rather than *created* societal expectations. As this pattern has been the case in society, so has it been evident in medicine.[1] Although many benefits have accrued for women and doctors since the nineteenth century, feminist researchers, whether espousing passive or active views of women, point to areas in which medical treatments have often not been in women's best interests.

Doctors have many legitimate claims to job discontent. I concentrate here, however, more specifically on the woman patient. Although all women do not fit into one category, they do share common physiological processes. Different class, ethnic, racial, or individually grouped women, embedded as they are in diverse contexts, may define these processes differently. This sameness and difference allows for a unifying basis among women—shared experience with enormous variety. Yet all women in America, in some way, come in contact with biomedical definitions of women's bodies—definitions that assume a sameness separated from women's experiences. Women are treated individually for particular concerns but are conceptually lumped together in the generalized category of Woman. In this chapter I review the problems women face when reproductive needs and the medical system intersect.

BACKGROUND NOTES

Pudendum or *Pudenda:* also known as vulva from the Latin Pudere, "to be ashamed of."
Estrogen: from the Greek oistros, "insane desire."
Hysterectomy: from the Greek hysteria, "belonging to the womb."

Women and Language News, 1984

Irving Zola asserts that we all are at risk of becoming chronically ill or disabled. For 52 percent of the United States population, some would argue, that day starts at birth with the words "It's a girl." Modern Western society has historically conceptualized women as inferior, from the language used to describe female organs to the social and political theories of our culture, which are really about men. Examples from philosophers such as Aristotle—women are constitutionally unfitted for public life—to Rousseau—"It is of men that I am to speak" (in Okin 1979)—to modern psychological theories about development—"In the life cycle, as in the Garden of Eden, the woman has been the deviant" (Gilligan 1982)—the focus has been on males as the norm: "'Human nature,' we realize, as described and discovered by philosophers such as Aristotle, Aquinas, Machiavelli, Locke, Rousseau, Hegel, and many others, is intended to refer only to male human nature. Consequently, all the rights and needs that they have considered humanness to entail have not been perceived as applicable to the female half of the human race" (Okin 1979:6–7).

Women are theoretically conceptualized as deviant. This ideological thread runs through our institutions down to daily practices, which, in turn, reinforce these more abstract theoretical assumptions.

Medical institutions, too, share this heritage. Starting in the eighteenth century, and culminating in medicalization by the twentieth century, women's physiology has undergone definitional shifts. Each reproductive phase of women's lives is defined as a pathological condition in need of expert, medical, usually male, control (Rothman 1982, Todd 1983).[2] The male body is the norm. Women's bodies have been conceptualized as deviations from this norm. Nineteenth-century medical views of women's physiology present a dreary picture indeed.

> Under the influence of the female sexual organs, the strong characteristically become weak; fickleness supervenes upon a judgment previously calm and clear; indecision upon resolution; pusillanimity upon fearlessness and courage; deceitfulness upon a frank, open manner. We believe that the habits of truth-telling and fidelity in the social and domestic relations are more frequently broken up by irritable ovaries than by a native tendency to depravity in the female sex. Here, for example, is a young lady with an irritable ovary, who previously was fond of kittens, but who now falls into a swoon at the sight of one; then, here is another lady who was formerly very fond of society, but who now, from a familiar cause, has a dread of it, and prefers solitude; then again, another, who for the same proximate reasons, dislikes, repels, and finally leaves, the man she has solemnly sworn to love. (Gorton 1890:228–29)

In 1866, Dr. Isaac Ray stated: "With woman it is but a step from extreme nervous susceptibility to downright hysteria, and from that to overt insanity. In the sexual evolution, in pregnancy, in the parturient period, in lactation, strange thoughts, extraordinary feelings, unseasonable appetites, criminal impulses, may haunt a mind at other times innocent and pure" (Ray 1866:267).

Surgical procedures were used as remedies for these disorders. Women were first defined as deviant by their behavior and then in turn this deviance was attributed to their biology, requiring medical intervention. The reproductive organs became the primary focus for this intervention, whether the problem was defined as physical, mental, or moral. Removal of the uterus—"what she is in health, in character, in her charms, alike of body, mind and soul is because of her womb alone" (Storer 1871:79)—came to be viewed as an acceptable procedure for treating psychological, sexual, and physiological disorders. Castration and sexual surgery such as clitoridectomy were diagnoses for such "disorders" as masturbation or a "heightened" interest in sex, or such "sins" as using contraceptives and abortion. Removal of the ovaries was thought to cure insanity and excessive interest in sex—the two often being equated. Debates raged among doctors as to the efficacy, not to mention humaneness, of such treatments, but the results were that as women became more accustomed to male doctors, their health care increasingly revolved around surgical procedures. This was particularly true among the middle and upper classes. Just as some women actively rebelled against the strict sanctions of society in various movements and individual actions, others sought out the new medical practices. Sexual surgery became fashionable (see Scull and Favreau 1986)—perhaps sought by women out of boredom, anxiety for health, or to relieve weaknesses that had become self-fulfilling prophecies—a cure for all that was said to be wrong in a woman.

Many women yearning for improvements in basic health and reproductive control also turned to the new medical men as new technologies arose. They sought such improvements as painless childbirth or effective birth control as means to increase control over their lives (Riessman 1983). At times women, especially affluent women, pursued their own class interests at the expense of poorer women's rights. Innovations such as forceps promised doctors a technological edge and attracted wealthy women with the lure of safer, easier birth. Both doctors and women turned hopefully to the new techniques despite little evidence of promises fulfilled.[3] Thus it can be argued that women were participants in the medical acquisition of reproductive care. When women shared in medical change, however, they did so in a context they did not create. Women, anxious for safer, less painful childbirth, turned to those who promised it, actively seeking an end to biological destiny. Women were thus active but not equal participants in the medicalization of reproduction.[4]

Medical control is the practical consequence of this long and complex history of medicalization (Ehrenreich and English 1978, Gordon 1976, Leavitt 1984, Smith-Rosenberg and Rosenberg 1984, and Wertz and Wertz 1977 are some of the scholars to explore these complexities). This control has led to an overdependence on doctors by women—a reliance that is in turn used to prove women weak. First women were encouraged to turn to doctors for all their needs. As they increasingly did so, they were, and have continued to be, criticized for such dependence.

Today discrimination toward women, pervasive in our society, is also deeply embedded in the field of medicine. Doctors are in a unique position vis-à-vis women. They are the major source of information and treatment of women's reproductive processes—processes that embody serious decisions and carry culturally laden stereotypes. Whereas nineteenth-century women were defined as invalid because of their wombs, today twentieth-century women are defined more subtly—for example, they are often assumed to be disabled because of their hormones. The medical profession, though not the main creator of these attitudes, does play an important role in the reinforcement of societal assumptions about women. The reproductive cycle, from menstruation to menopause, is treated in a disease-oriented medical model by a surgeon.

Feminist scholarship has undertaken the difficult task of reconceptualizing reproduction—a reconceptualization that seeks understanding based on women's experiences rather than society's definitions. Reproductive cycles are redefined as healthy and ongoing experiences in women's daily lives. This is not to deny the very real physiological experiences that do often accompany women's cycles such as premenstrual changes, morning sickness, hot flashes, problems associated with high-risk pregnancies, and so forth, or the need for ongoing contraceptive research. But to turn the routine biology of half the population into diseases exaggerates the problem and stigmatizes women. It can also make them sicker. Once reproductive processes are defined as diseased, the door is open to overuse of interventionary procedures.[5]

In other words, doctors and women patients bring very different views of women's bodies to medical encounters. Birth control decisions, for example, are extremely complex in the making and in the consequences. Nevertheless, in the doctor's office, contraceptive choices are usually the end result of a brief physical exam and a short discussion of a contraceptive method(s). When the pros and cons of various contraceptive methods are discussed, they usually revolve around such issues as "risk factors" and "efficacy records." When the physical exam is completed and birth control options are reviewed, the contraceptive "choice" is usually a prescription.[6] For doctors, women's bodies are just that—physiological parts to be cured, changed, and controlled (with problems in some cases seen as psychogenic in origin).

To define these decisions so narrowly in the medical model limits women's control and role in the decision-making process. It also obscures the complexities involved. For example, at home in daily life birth control decisions and use are much more than a medical topic. They take place in a broader context that can include relationships, religious influences, sexuality, family dynamics, and economic considerations, as well as physiological concerns. For women to separate their bodies from who they are in the larger context of their lives is like trying to separate two sides of a coin.[7]

Despite a less than perfect fit, the medical system is committed to continued control of reproductive care. It is a system organized around and dependent on women as patients: the majority of drugs are prescribed largely to women; women are the most frequent visitors to the doctor whether for themselves or their families, and obstetrician-gynecologists are one of the highest paid specialists in medicine, with women making up all of their clientele. The diseasing of reproduction heralded a new age for medical men, providing, whether premeditated or not, a large, lucrative, and continuous patient population (Ehrenreich and English 1978, Luker 1984, Todd 1983, Wertz and Wertz 1977).[8]

The gradual shift in perceptions of reproduction during the late nineteenth and early twentieth centuries from social/organic, female-controlled normal functions to biological/technological, male-controlled disease processes is today firmly entrenched in our assumptions and institutions (Merchant 1980). Women live in the same world as doctors and share cultural assumptions that perpetuate these relationships. Society's values, though part of the background context, often go unexamined by people in their daily lives. Unless something disrupts us, our actions are often routine. We do not in each instance of action or interaction unravel these background assumptions. Doctors do not say to themselves, "I want to control the care of this woman's body," and women do not say, "My well body is in danger of being treated in a disease model." When seen in this light, the diseasing of women is neither the sole creation of medical practices nor that of women's strivings. Rather, doctors' interactions with women and women's with doctors reflect and reinforce the prevailing views in our society (to be discussed further in Chapter 5).

History, culture, and societal views have a direct bearing on medical practices. But what does this mean for doctors and patients? What are medical encounters like? Interactions neither occur in a vacuum nor are they wholly determined by societal norms. Rather, a dialectic relationship exists in which daily events in people's lives both influence and are influenced by the larger society and culture. Medical interactions bear witness to the intricacies of these connections. To understand better women's daily experiences of their reproductive processes and the medical care they receive, social scientists have focused recently on interactions between practitioners and female patients. Ironically, today, it seems that this once-so-compliant (perhaps only seemingly) population is the most dissatisfied with its medical care. Although the literature is small, it provides essential information about the dynamics of this relationship.

WHEN THE PATIENT IS A WOMAN

A doctor who remembers that his patient has his own mantle of dignity—which is admittedly not easy to think about a naked person clutching a sheet and wearing an alarmed expression—will not be patronizing in his form of address. He will not call patients by their first names while expecting to have his own title used and he will not object to explaining what he means when it is not clear to someone whose education has been in a different field. Column note [Miss Manners']: You will note that Miss Manners has used the pronoun *he* about offending doctors. This is because she has noticed women doctors who have behaved better. They may be a statistical error. (Miss Manners, *Washington Post*, March 9, 1980)

Miss Manners's advice to doctors is an example of the widespread interest in the doctor-patient relationship. It is also an example of how difficult it is to overcome cultural accoutrements. For though Miss Manners carefully explains her use of the male pronoun for the doctor, the male usage for the patient remains unexamined (line 1).

The majority of doctor-patient relationships are still between male doctors and female patients. First, by the end of 1986 only 15.2 percent of doctors were women with even fewer female gynecologists. Although this proportion is changing, the effects of large numbers of women doctors on medical care are still unknown. Second, women go to doctors more than men. Why they do so has been a source of argument for some time. The traditional rationale has been that women are the weaker, more sickly sex. There are other explanations. Women, because of their general socialization, are more likely to seek help, to be able to admit a problem. Furthermore, Linda Fidell (in Schiefelbein 1980) points out that when women's longer life span is controlled for, the figures for sickness become more equal between the sexes. Whatever the explanation, the major consumers of health care, whether for themselves or for their families, are women.

As discussed in the last chapter, many pressures on doctors and on patients contribute to a subtle adversarial relationship. People feel more powerless in unfamiliar surroundings, a feeling complicated by the stress of illness and the elevated status of the doctor. When the patient is a woman, the scenario becomes even more complex.

The Complaining Patient

Medical training has been criticized for educating students in how to play God. This medical socialization has also influenced students in how to think of women patients. "Critics of physician training note that physicians have been systematically schooled in the belief that women are inferior, are less competent, present psychosomatic complaints and are hysterical" (Jansen, 1987:250). These attitudes, still present in current texts, can become translated into medical practice.

Research findings show female patients being taken less seriously than male patients. Gena Corea (1977) reports that when doctors were asked to describe a "typical complaining patient," 72 percent referred to a woman, 4 percent to a man. Karen Armitage and colleagues (1979) examined 104 charts of men and women with non-sex-specific complaints—back pain, headache, dizziness, chest pain, and fatigue. They found medical work-ups for the men to be significantly more detailed than those for the women, suggesting that men's problems were given more credence.

During medical interviews the discourse patterns disclose similar findings. Wallen and associates (1979) found that doctors answered male patients' technical questions with equivalently sophisticated answers more easily than those of women. Women were more likely to be talked down to even when they asked knowledgeable questions. John McKinlay's (1975) article "Who Is Really Ignorant?" complements these data, discussing how male doctors systematically underestimate women's abilities to understand medical terms, diagnoses, and so forth, encouraging a patronizing manner toward the patient. Although it is important that doctors be clear and avoid lapsing into medical jargon, it is equally crucial to avoid talking down to women as if they were well-meaning children.

It is this infantilization that women have so objected to in recent years. Despite lengthy discussions in the *New England Journal of Medicine* (over several editions) on the problems of addressing patients by their first names and expecting them to address the doctor by title, this is still the most common form of exchange. Such a minor example of medical dominance (and one so easy to rectify) seems to elude the majority of doctors. A more serious discourtesy to women patients, and perhaps not unconnected, has been the ongoing dismissal of their complaints as psychosomatic, overemotional responses, all in their heads.

The UCLA Department of Medicine (in Schiefelbein 1980) simulated cases on paper, stating the sex of the patient, with all problems organic in origin. They found doctors' diagnoses of women to be 30 percent more likely than men's to involve emotional factors and twice as likely to be labeled entirely emotional. Michele Barrett and Helen Roberts (1978) in a study of English general practitioners (with real patients) display similar findings. Doctors took men's illnesses as well as life stresses more seriously than women's. The men were viewed as hard workers in a competitive world—something the doctors themselves could relate to. Doctors tended to blame the social situation for men's problems. Women, on the other hand, were defined by doctors in terms of the family and home, being plagued by "vague and spurious worries" generally psychosomatic in origin. Doctors were less sympathetic, blaming the individual women rather than social arrangements for their "unfounded" aches and pains.

Such labeling invites diagnoses of depression and prescriptions for mood-altering drugs. Twice as many women as men are prescribed tranquilizers and barbiturates (Wolcott 1979), and prescription drug abuse, particularly among women, is a continuing social problem. General sentiment in society and in medicine often supports the notion that women have it easy, raising adorable tots and eating bonbons. This stereotype presents an unrealistic picture of women's lives. Women have always worked outside and inside the home, and their numbers in the paid work force are steadily increasing. Those who *are* full-time housewives usually find it a physically and mentally demanding job.

Jean Rhys, novelist and portrayor of sad ladies, captures this point in her short story "Outside the Machine." Mrs. Murphy has attempted suicide outside and is now inside the hospital, garnering little sympathy.

> It seemed they all knew about Mrs. Murphy. They knew that she had tried the same thing on before. Suddenly, by magic, they seemed to know all about her. And what a thing to do, to try to kill yourself! If it had been a man, now, you might have been a bit sorry. You might have said, "Perhaps the poor devil has had a rotten time." But a woman!
>
> "A married woman with two sweet little kiddies."
>
> "The fool," said Pat. "My God, what would you do with a fool like that?" . . .
>
> "She's one of these idiotic neurasthenics, neurotics, or whatever you call them. She says she's frightened of life, I ask you. That's why she's here. Under observation. . . ."
>
> "I'm so awfully sorry for her husband." . . . "And her children. So sorry. The poor kiddies, the poor sweet little kiddies. . . . Oughtn't a woman like that to be hung?"
>
> "What's she got to be neurasthenic and neurotic about anyway?" Pat demanded. "If she has a perfectly good husband and kiddies, what's she got to be neurasthenic and neurotic about?"
>
> Stone and iron, their voices were. One was stone and one was iron. (1960:106–7)

Research and literature both show that women run a greater risk than do men of being labeled overemotional when physically or mentally troubled. But what about when they go to doctors with obvious, clearly defined social and physiological needs such as pregnancy? Once again, though treated, some say overtreated, for this condition, the mental set is often the same. The Lennanes (1973) and Jarnfelt (1982) found that though the majority of women (70 to 88 percent) routinely suffer morning sickness during the early months of pregnancy, the medical literature abounds with the "real" meanings of such symptoms—neurotic immaturity, inability to cope with impending motherhood, and the general psychosomatic nature of women, to name a few. Women are first labeled as neurotic and then their biology is used to prove the point.

The term *psychosomatic* has a derogatory history, implying a malingerer, a willful patient who is sick needlessly. William Barclay in the *Journal of the American Medical Association* discusses in a telling statement the consequences of overlooking serious problems by being too eager to dismiss women's symptoms. "I think pain in women *is* more often psychogenic than organic. . . . [But] an organic problem is sometimes overlooked—not often—but when it happens it's a tragedy. An error in judgment could cost a life. You'll live with it forever. You can't accumulate too many penalties or you're out of the game" (in Schiefelbein 1980:14). Acknowledgment of connections between stress and disease, as well as Barclay's point, are well taken, but as long as doctors continue to define women's problems as "more often" psychogenically oriented, whether the diagnosis is taken more seriously or not the margin for error will be large. Doctors have to live with it forever, but so do patients, who run the risk of also finding themselves "out of the game."

The consequences of not taking women's descriptions seriously are movingly discussed by Marianne Paget (1983) in her article on medical misunderstandings. This is a case study of three visits between an internist and a recovering cancer patient in a university-affiliated clinic. Paget provides a detailed discourse analysis of a doctor who dismisses the patient's complaints as "nerves." On each visit the patient lists aspects of her health that are causing her pain and worry: (1) pain on scalp, (2) pain in mouth and teeth that interferes with her sleep ("my mouth is drivin me crazy" [p. 57]), (3) pain on surgery scar, (4) pain in kidney, trouble walking up stairs, overtired. The patient concludes that she has not had much stamina lately and is "not a happy person to be with" (p. 65), in contrast with a past description of herself as an active person. The doctor early in the relationship raises the issue of nerves: "W'll has it possibly occurred to you that with all the troubles that yer . . . body has gone through that yer nerves *have now got* to the point where they suffer an where you need help to get yer nerves restored" (p. 67).

In conclusion, Paget points out that nowhere in the three interviews did the topic of this patient's experiences with cancer come up for discussion—how she was feeling about it, coping with the experience, and so forth. The doctor's diagnosis of "nerves" came up early and flavored all of the discourse regarding her health. The patient's agitation and nervousness over her condition further confirmed his assessment of her complaints as emotional in nature. During these discussions, the doctor continually interrupted the patient, changing topics and redirecting them to confirm further his diagnosis of postoperative nerves and depression. Although one could argue that this doctor delivered poor medicine by diagnosing the patient as nervous and then sending her home to take care of herself without offering advice, referral, or even a chance to talk about her reactions, the real outcome is indeed the tragedy Barclay speaks of. This patient, seeking care at another hospital, reported that she was diagnosed as having cancer of the spine that had been present but had remained undetected by her internist.

A Difference in Perspective

So far in this chapter I have reviewed available research to examine medical attitudes toward women patients—the fact that they are on one hand squeezed into a biomedical model and on the other hand they are sometimes not taken seriously, defined as overemotional malingerers. These attitudes are learned by all the participants from an early age, first from society and then in medical school, and are later reenacted in health care delivery. Surely one might ask, Don't some women have health problems that are considered "real"? All women going to all doctors cannot be dismissed as psychosomatically driven. This is, of course, the case. Women go to doctors for reproductive care involving birth control and pregnancy, for diseases such as cancer or appendicitis, or for chronic ailments for which their concerns *are* taken seriously. Research in this area highlights another set of problems—the patient's perspective is not always the same as the doctor's, and this can cause problems for both. "Doctors and patients can be said to hold very different models of reality as a result of their socialization into dominant-subordinant roles, which usually also follow male-female lines" (Romalis in Treichler and Kramarae 1984). Cristina Cacciari (1984) in a study of Italian gynecologist-patient communication concluded that the two talked in different modes. The former inclined toward a direct question-answer style, with the latter trying to insert a broader, storytelling mode. The doctors usually dominated the conversation, thus cutting off the patients' contributions. The setting is ripe for misunderstandings and dissatisfactions, with the doctor finding the patient difficult to communicate with (reinforcing already held prejudices) and the patient feeling cut off and inadequate.

Hilary Graham and Ann Oakley, in their English study of pregnant women and obstetricians, found conflict of perspective to be a fundamental feature in this relationship, whether or not the participants were aware of it. "We are suggesting that doctors and mothers have a qualitatively different way of looking at the nature, context and management of reproduction" (1981:51). Doctors view pregnant women through a biomedical model that defines them as patients and pregnancy as an isolated medical event. Women view this event as a holistic, integrated part in the larger context of their lives. It is not hard to imagine these women trying to talk to their doctors in the storytelling style Cacciari found in her research while the physicians assume a question-answer format. In studying this discourse between mothers and doctors, Graham and Oakley highlight a conflict that is won by doctors, influencing maternity care and delivery. An example from their data finds an expectant mother being told she will need the baby induced (labor will be started in the hospital by a drug). She has stated that she does not "fancy that very much" and goes on to probe a reluctant doctor.

> *Patient:* If my husband wanted to come and talk to you about inducing me, can I make an appointment for him?
> *Doctor:* I don't think anything your husband said would affect our decision one way or the other.
> *Patient:* No, but he would like to talk to you.
> *Doctor:* Yes, well he can talk to whoever's on duty, but there's nothing he can say that will affect us: it's a medical question. . . . I think you've got to assume if you come here for medical attention that we make all the decisions. (pp. 62–63)

Overt disagreement was rare in these interactions. It was to the researchers that the women commonly reported their dissatisfactions with the care they were receiving:

  (a) not feeling able to ask questions;

  (b) not having sufficient explanation of medical treatment or the progress of the pregnancy from the doctor;

  (c) being treated as ignorant;

  (d) seeing too many different doctors;

  (e) feeling rushed, like "battery hens," animals in a "cattle market" or items on a "conveyor belt" or an "assembly line." (pp. 63–64)

This research is from England, but it sounds similar to complaints from clinic patients in this country—the time is too short, the doctor too rushed, continuity of care is lacking, doctors talk too much and do not listen enough.[9]

Doris Betts's fiction provides a poignant picture of women's experiences. Her story of a young woman's alienated birth describes what it can feel like when birth is treated as a medical event—an event marked here, in the end, by attitudes toward women's sexuality. Gwen is on the delivery table after a long and confusing labor.

> He [the doctor] explained she would be able to bear down, by will, even though she would notice only the intent to do so, and not feel herself pushing. So when they said bear down, Gwen thought about that, and somebody else bore down somewhere to suit them.
> "High forceps." Two hands molded something below her navel, outside, and pressed it.
> "Now" . . .
> Suddenly the doctor was very busy and, like a magician, tugged out of nowhere a long and slimy blue-gray thing, one gut spilling from its tail. No that was the cord, umbilical cord. He dropped the mass wetly on the sheet near Gwen's waist. . . . Then that blunt end of it rolled, became a face, bas relief, carved shallow on one side. The mouth gave a sickly mew and, before her eyes, the whole length began to bleach and to pinken. Gwen could hardly breathe from watching while it lay loosely on her middle. . . . The baby screamed and shook a fist wildly at the great surgical light. . . . He [the doctor] finished with the cord, handed the baby to a man in a grocer's apron. . . .
> The pediatrician she and Richard had chosen was already busy at another table. Cleaning him, binding him, piling him into a scale for weight. Dr. Somers explained that Gwen must lie perfectly flat in bed, no pillow, so the spinal block would not give her headaches. . . . [later] Gwen tried to sit up but a nun leaned on her shoulder. "Flat on your back, Mrs. Gower."
> "I want to see."
> "Shh."

The doctor finishes up the birth by stitching the episiotomy.

> "A small incision so you wouldn't be torn by the birth. An episiotomy. I'll take the stitches now." Dr. Somers winked between her knees. "Some women ask me to take an extra stitch to tighten them for their husband."
> Stitch up the whole damn thing, Gwen thought. (1975:279–80)

Gwen is silent, but her thoughts are vivid. Women, in real life or in fiction, may have doubts about their treatment, but, for the most part, they do not express their reservations to medical staff.

Negotiations Between Doctors and Patients

Sue Fisher (1986) found that in the rare cases when patients' reservations were expressed, treatment outcomes were affected. She studied cervical cancer in two clinics—a faculty clinic serving middle- and upper-class patients referred from private physicians and treated regularly by the same staff physician, and the community clinic serving lower-class, poorer patients referred by local clinics and treated by rotating residents. Doctors' power in her data could be seen in their presentations of information to patients. The community clinic patients ran a higher risk of hysterectomy than did women in the faculty clinic even when they had exactly the same symptoms and medical assessments. She asserts that these treatment decisions are reached through strategic negotiations between doctors and patients in which linguistic strategies assume great importance. Her findings show residents persuading patients to have hysterectomies even when there were less invasive procedures available. Patients who used questioning techniques, however, could trigger the provider to list alternatives, thus avoiding a hysterectomy. Straightforward questions such as "Is a hysterectomy necessary?" or as one woman asked nervously and even incomprehensively, "Have a hysterectomy and that, I'm that, if there's an alternative" (p. 51), influenced treatment outcomes. Given the increase in asymmetry between doctors and patients when social class is involved, it becomes all the more crucial that women of all classes and races have access to communication strategies for negotiating medical decisions.

Most recommendations for improving doctor-patient communication have focused on changing medical training, giving workshops in hospitals, and so forth. This is, indeed, important. Less experimented with but equally important is educating patients in navigating the medical setting and interview. As Fisher is careful to point out, communication techniques and education will not end all the problems that plague this relationship. But she shows in her work that it is important for women to learn the right questions to ask in the hope of gaining more control over their health care.

Women have begun, in fact, in small numbers to question their doctors, making demands that in the past were unthought of. Self-help health books (most notably *Our Bodies, Ourselves*) abound, and the women's health movement has developed a wide array of informational resources for patient education. Patients are becoming more knowledgeable and in turn wanting more information about their choices, about drugs prescribed, and about their doctors' recommendations. Although undoubtedly many doctors respond to this questioning well, encouraging more active participation by their patients, what little data we have show that doctors can also find it a threat to their power. Barrett and Roberts (1978) found in England that doctors wanted patients to be recipients of knowledge from the expert (themselves) rather than equal participants in their health care.

Symonds (1983), a New York psychiatrist, suggests that while women are slowly becoming more informed and less passive in doctor-patient interviews, doctors are becoming defensive and see the questioning of their procedures as challenges to their authority. She concludes, first, that doctors are used to power and that power equals status and money, neither of which they want to lose. Second, the assertive, knowledgeable woman does not mesh with societal expectations and stereotypes, which many people, doctors being no exception, still hold despite current changes. The well-informed patient can cause the doctor anxiety leading to defensiveness. In turn, Mary Jansen points out that people's behavior is influenced by how they are treated and perceived. "If women are seen as more helpless, dependent, and passive than men, this may encourage them to present themselves as anxious and depressed in order to fit expected sex-role stereotypes" (1987:3). The cycle is hard to break. Some women go to the doctor and behave as expected, reinforcing the doctor's conventional image of women patients. Better-informed patients may attempt to establish a more equal relationship, only to find that they receive a double dose of medical management and become labeled difficult.

Silent Rebellion

This chapter was introduced with women's comments about doctors. Their statements were hostile and critical. The diseasing of reproduction provides fertile grounds for such dissatisfaction. In my data, from two medical settings, most women had something negative to say about their health care in general and/or doctors in particular. My findings are supported by the studies mentioned above. Given historical and current approaches to women's health in the United States (and the Western world), such attitudes are not surprising. What is surprising, however, are the doctor-patient interactions. In my transcripts, as well as in the observed interactions and reviewed literature, friendly, submissive behavior on the part of women was the rule, not the exception. Hostility was expressed to the researchers, not the doctors. Although patient assertiveness is growing, it is still rare. Dissatisfaction, when expressed, was shown by silence and withdrawal, which are difficult to define as displeasure without a follow-up interview. Where were the assertive "yucks," and "bullshit," and "rip-off artists" or at least detailed questioning of recommended procedures? They were veiled in polite responses to doctors' initiatives, all fitting the medical ideals of "good patients." In fact, the attending doctors were unaware of this unstated skepticism about medical care.

Although women may be in a passive role in doctors' offices, they appear to take an active role in their health care once outside of these offices. Women are more likely to change their doctors than are men (Lavin 1983), and though there are no specific data, my discussions with alternative medical practitioners suggest that women more than men turn to unconventional methods of healing. A complicated picture of the relationship between doctor and female patient emerges. In sum, women use medical care more than men, perhaps because of a more help-oriented socialization and their need of health services for reproductive care as well as disease. The literature just discussed illustrates that in seeking this care, women report many dissatisfactions. There is no evidence, however, that these dissatisfactions are voiced to doctors. In fact, women's complaints, in general, seem to take the form of silent rebellion, such as noncompliance and changing practitioners, rather than direct confrontation.

Several factors contribute to the dynamic in this relationship. Medical dominance, for example, inhibits direct confrontation. Patients share the same world view and socialization as doctors—a view that assumes the doctor knows best. Although people may question this outside the office, they are less sure once in the doctor's domain. The position of doctors as well-meaning, in a healing, helping role, makes it seem inappropriate for a patient to question their help. All of the above could apply to all patients, men or women. What, then, makes the doctor–female patient relationship unique? In this chapter, I have reviewed research that examines why doctors treat women differently from how they treat men. But how do we understand why women participate in the manner described above? Contributions from recent developmental psychological theories can be useful in illuminating why women may be so compliant in the doctor-patient relationship.

Carol Gilligan's (1982) reformulation of moral development in males and females is a case in point. She starts with Lawrence Kohlberg's (1981) stages of human development, reevaluating exactly what this process means for women. Kohlberg has delineated six progessive stages of moral development, starting with childhood and ending with adult maturity. He developed these universal levels from a twenty-year study of eighty-four males, and when he applied these stages to females he found women to be deficient. Women's development stopped at stage three—the interpersonal level at which goodness equals pleasing others—rather than reaching the levels of the understanding of general rules over interpersonal relationships (stage four) and culminating in universal principles of justice (stages five and six) equivalent to full maturity, found in male development. Female moral development centered on self-sacrifice and responsibility to others at the interpersonal level with a general focus on relationships. Men develop a hierarchical, universal definition of right; women's sense of right is contextual and relational.

At face value such a theoretical framework would contribute to my data on women's actions. One could argue that women's development into such an interpersonally other-directed model would lead to "good-girl" behavior, especially in the less familiar surroundings of the medical setting, perhaps undressed in the presence of a nonintimate, usually male doctor. Although there is a grain of truth in this, women are left in a blame-the-victim position of (1) inadequate development leading to (2) immaturity, resulting in (3) inability to interact responsibly and equally in society.

Gilligan has taken all of this and turned it on its head. First, she has criticized Kohlberg's premises, pointing out that to discuss theories of universal human development from a study of males is geared to make men the norm. This fits with general social theories, as well as the medical attitudes toward women discussed earlier. It bolsters the status quo yet does not fully inform us about the complexities of gender difference and human behavior.

The studies by Gilligan and her colleagues reevaluate both male and female development, looking at the differences and how they can present costs and benefits for each sex as well as for society. In testing male and female college students, Gilligan found that men's fears arise from close personal ties and intimacy. Men appear to feel safer in impersonal, more objective, success-oriented situations. Women believe just the opposite—safety lies in closeness and the interpersonal, danger in the risk of aloneness. Women will strive for connection, men for separation. Gilligan criticizes each pole as too narrow—women are socialized to be too self-sacrificing and other-oriented within relationships, while men become too detached and self-focused.

Gilligan's findings reflect limited roles for both sexes but are especially damaging for women, because the male scale is considered normal. Women can thus find themselves in a double bind—if they fit the female version, they are dismissed as immature, dependent, overemotional, just one easy step away from hysterical; but if they try to break down these stereotypes, they are seen as trying to be men, denying their natural selves.

Gilligan calls for a reinterpretation of women's skills. Rather than defining women as developmentally disadvantaged based on their interpersonal abilities, she argues that these abilities enhance people's lives. Although Gilligan provides a more positive vision of women, her vision is in other ways no less problematic than Kohlberg's. For Gilligan, women, by implication all women, develop in essentially the same way, and it is the individual internal development that for her lies at the base of women's interactional style. In other words, when the patient is a woman, the interaction is different because she *is* a woman. But the problem lies not so much in women's development as in the value, or lack of it, that society places on their development—a devaluation of the feminine that is internalized by the men and women who become doctors and the women who are patients.

CONCLUSION

A society's values develop historically and are deeply embedded in institutional arrangements and individual consciousness. Doctors and patients bring to their interactions complex internalizations of larger societal expectations. Physicians carry with them assumptions about women which have been nurtured for many generations and are difficult to change even in these times of increasing awareness. Discussion of doctors' reactions to assertive women in the medical office bears this out. On one hand, doctors have long complained about the overemotional nature of their female patients, and on the other, when faced with confident women, they can become defensive. Many women bring with them the socialization to be "good girls," to make sure that the conversation is pleasant, regardless of how they feel, and to try to establish an interpersonal relationship in their interactions. This can be particularly true in situations with people defined as authorities.

This latter point is particularly relevant here. All patients go to the doctor and are squeezed into a scientific model that separates the mind from the body/organ/cell, reducing the person to the disease or condition. People of both sexes have complained about this situation vigorously, and the model needs to be broadened. The hierarchical organization of medicine presents another model men and women face when seeking health care. Doctors are assumed to be the dominant figure with patients playing a subordinate role. Patients are supposed to be docile. But women also go to the doctor in the context of a male model that demands detached behavior from a population largely socialized and encouraged to be interpersonally conscious and skilled. Thus we see the patients in Cacciari's study trying unsuccessfully to tell stories that incorporate their health and their lives, while the doctors orchestrate question-answer sequences, and in Graham and Oakley's observations that pregnant women want to contextualize their conditions, which to the doctors, who control the occasions, are cut-and-dried biological events. These daily interactions are embedded in a long history of attitudes and practices toward women that are glaringly apparent to the trained eye but so assumed as to be nearly undetectable to those less aware. The scientific approach that separates biology from social context, the male role that encourages detachment and distance, societal attitudes toward women, and the hierarchical arrangements that provide doctors with the power to implement these usually unexamined perspectives combine to create a daunting, complicated scenario for women patients.

Women's abilities to express their feelings, tell their stories, and establish rapport have been systematically denied in modern medical practice. This situation may be acceptable to the doctor in the interaction, but it is not necessarily pleasing to the woman. Rather than dismissing women's emotions and broader contextual understandings of health and illness, these responses could be redefined in such a way as to enrich the medical model, reconceptualize male-female and doctor-patient relationships, and improve health care delivery. Doctors and patients do not need to sit for hours commiserating and swapping personal life stories, but rather to garner new respect for an old tradition—women's ability to tell their stories in an atmosphere in which problems are discussed cooperatively, rather than one in which an expert treats a passive patient. Medical care for women and for men would improve. As Ingelfinger has suggested, "The doctor who treats a woman badly is apt to treat all patients badly" (in Schiefelbein 1980).

NOTES

1. This pattern is observable today in feminist critiques of reproductive technologies. In the late 1960s, when women began questioning their lives as mothers and wives, they rejected motherhood as their primary role. Women were responding against society's pressures. Today, as childbirth and motherhood are in danger more and more of becoming technological events controlled by male doctors and scientists (see Arditti et al. 1984), feminist writers, in an effort to alert women to this threat, have at times romanticized motherhood. Once again, women find themselves responding to social forces in an ongoing struggle to have some control over their lives and to live in a better society. Before one wall is scaled, another higher, thicker wall is in place.

2. The majority of doctors today are men, and there are even fewer women in gynecology than in general medical practices. Although this situation is changing with more women going to medical school and into gynecology, it is too soon to know whether this will bring about fundamental change.

3. Throughout the history of technological innovation there are examples of new techniques that have brought great promise and swept people up in the excitement, only to be later cast aside or changed beyond recognition. Forceps, originally quite large and cumbersome and we now know dangerous, have been remodeled time and time again. Today, rather than being used in the average birth, they are recommended for use only in difficult births.

4. This is an important and easily misunderstood point. Just because women were active participants in the social construction of the diseasing of reproduction, they should not be blamed for their own oppression—a danger in this argument. To say that women were equal participants in this medicalization is analogous to the claim that blacks liked slavery because, when freed, some returned or stayed on the plantations. Rather, in both cases, it is an issue of coerced will when the choices were limited.

5. An example of how dangerous the diseasing of reproduction is for women's health is the high and widely criticized hysterectomy rate. Diana Scully (1980) reports that surgery rates, in general, have been growing in the United States, but hysterectomies have undergone a particularly dramatic rise. In the early 1970s, hysterectomy was the fourth most frequently performed operation. Between 1970 and 1975, the hysterectomy rate rose 24 percent and is now the most frequently performed operation. It is estimated that over half the U.S. female population will have some form of hysterectomy before the age of sixty-five. Although some of these

surgeries certainly save lives and improve health, many are seen as unnecessary, jeopardizing health and lives.

6. Birth control pills are the number one *prescribed* method of contraception in the United States. Sterilization, both male and female, however, is the most used method of birth control.

7. Women are at risk when birth control is treated exclusively as a health issue, but ironically the risks are also great when it is *not* seen as one. On one hand, medical experts have the cultural authority to define the parameters of health. Since reproduction is defined in this category, birth control is treated in an acontextual model which ignores women's life experiences. On the other hand, birth control in our society is embedded in various moralisms and subject to the law—not a health issue and thus not in any way a right. Women's ability to make a choice is thus influenced by medical, societal, and cultural influences that often go unexamined and are at times in conflict with each other, beyond women's control.

Rosalind Petchesky (1985) makes a similar argument about abortion. Women's reproduction is too exclusively defined as a health issue. Women seeking reproductive care are locked into the medical model with all its attendant problems. But when women need access to birth control or abortion, such access is not considered a right, as having a broken leg set would be. Its health status is denied.

The question becomes how to define reproductive processes so that women will be able to find the help they need but maintain control over their bodies (as well as cultural definitions of their bodies). Petchesky argues that reproduction *is* a health issue and should be considered one; it is our understanding of health that needs to be changed. One suggestion is that reproductive care include respect for both "medical knowledge" and "individuals' life choices" (p. 168). She also suggests linking health needs to justice, justice implying "social, economic, and sexual needs; and needs are understood as the measure of rights" (p. 169). Such ideas are foreign to our present way of thinking about reproduction or health and are certainly absent in our medical system.

8. This is not to say that there were no genuine medical innovations that contributed to these changes. By the late nineteenth century, scientific advances in anesthesia and surgical techniques were gaining momentum. It is important to reiterate, however, that the changes in control of women's health care were started before there was any scientific basis for such a change.

9. Hospital versus home births have been debated in modern America as they were at the turn of the century. The American Medical Association (AMA) has argued that hospital births are safer than out-of-hospital births. When babies are born in taxis, ghetto backstairs, or bathrooms, his assertion is undoubtedly true. In studies comparing prepared home births with hospital births, however, the home is a perfectly safe place to give birth and, in fact, appears to be safer than hospitals for the non-high-risk delivery (Mehl 1977). Rothman (1982) in her book on childbirth in America depicts two models of labor and delivery. First, women being delivered in the medical model are just that—delivered. They are put in a passive position to be recipients of expert care. Control resides with the doctor and hospital. Second and in direct opposition to this approach is the midwifery model. Midwives help women birth their own babies, in their own time, in their own homes, under their own control. Whereas the doctor is the manager in the medical model, the midwife lends assistance to the birthing woman (and her chosen attendants) in the midwifery model.

3 | "The Patient Doesn't Have Anything to Say About It"

Doctor: Where is the drape [cloth used to cover women patients during a gynecological pelvic examination]?
Nurse: She did not want one.
Patient: I don't like them.
Doctor: [to the nurse] The patient doesn't have anything to say about it. She's going to use one. She might bleed and get everything about, uh, on her clothes, then she's going to squawk.
Nurse: Okay.
Doctor: [to the patient] In this office we always use a drape. Honey, maybe you'll start bleeding. You're going to soil your clothes and everything else.[1]

Sandra Kerry (the patient) has decided that being draped makes her feel alienated from the procedures done to her body and that she should be ashamed of her body. She has refused to use a drape on this visit. The nurse, surprised but compliant, puts the drape away. The doctor, a gynecologist in private practice, enters the examining room, sees the undraped patient, and demands that she follow his procedures in his office. Sandra Kerry complies.

Patient: It won't hurt, will it?
Doctor: Oh, I doubt it.
Patient: I'm taking your word (laugh).
Doctor: I haven't had anybody pass out from one yet [IUD].
Patient: The last time/
Doctor: (cuts patient off with a joke, both laugh)
Patient: The last time when I had that Lippes Loop, oh God/
Doctor: (interrupts patient)/You won't even know what's going on, we'll just slip that in and you'll be so busy talking and you won't know it.

Maria Martinez has come to the clinic for a pre-IUD (intrauterine device) examination. She has had an IUD in the past and is nervous about trying one again. She attempts to raise the topic of pain three times. On two of these attempts the doctor interrupts her efforts by providing her with information based on *his* assumption that she is concerned with pain *during* insertion of the IUD. But she is trying to raise a question based on *her* experience of pain *after* insertion. Since this exchange took place as the doctor was preparing to leave, he ended the interview unaware that Maria Martinez's question went unanswered and her contraceptive concerns and options unexplored.

In Chapters 1 and 2 I have drawn on diverse literatures to portray a broad picture of the doctor-patient relationship. In the next two chapters I turn to my own study of gynecologists and women patients in the examining room to provide more detailed analysis of medical relationships.

American women regularly visit gynecologists to ask questions about their reproductive processes. Because the two individuals, doctor and patient, have different concerns, the interaction becomes a negotiated process. People such as Maria Martinez initiate the medical relationship by seeking health care; yet ironically, in medical interactions the doctor dominates the discourse in the interview, not simply its diagnostic outcome. Thomas Scheff discusses this negotiation between psychiatrist and client, acknowledging the active participation of both parties but emphasizing the inequality of power between the doctors and clients:

> The interrogator's definition of the situation plays an important part in the joint definition of the situation which is finally negotiated. Moreover, his definition is more important than the client's in determining the final outcome of the negotiation, principally because he is well trained, secure, and self-confident in his role in the transaction, whereas the client is untutored, anxious and uncertain about his role in the transaction. Stated simply, the subject, because of these conditions is likely to be susceptible to the influence of the interrogator. (1968:6)

Scheff's point is observable in the research discussed in earlier chapters and in the data I collected on contraceptive and reproductive care. The discussion thus far has included varying levels of analysis to see medical relationships more clearly, especially when the patient is a woman. My purpose in this chapter is to look closely at the actual discourse of women talking with their doctors. A central theme in this chapter is power and how it is manifested in conversations between doctors and patients. This power has several faces. In some cases, as above with Maria Martinez, the doctor's dominance arises from a difference in assumptions and an un-awareness that this difference needs to be explored. Both parties are well-meaning, in this case friendly and joking with each other. Nonetheless, the necessary information does not get communicated, and the doctor slights the woman's concerns—not from wickedness, or even insensitivity, but rather from a confidence that he has gotten all the information he needs from her, has given her all the information she needs, and now has the knowledge to proceed. Other examples of medical dominance take a more obvious turn with the doctor consciously believing that it is his role to be in charge and the patient, like Sandra Kerry, indeed having nothing to say about it.

THE STUDY

Research for this study was conducted in a large American city over a two-and-one-half-year period. Two settings were observed. The first, a women's clinic, part of a community health center in a multicultural neighborhood, was a member of a nineteen-clinic network serving the city and suburbs. The clinic was staffed by a women's health care specialist, volunteers, and gynecological residents (doctors in specialty training) from two nearby training hospitals. The residents worked in the clinic, on the average, for one or two years and were paid by the hour. During my two years of re-search in the clinic, two residents were the primary health care providers. Both completed their residencies and left the clinic to establish their own practices as my research ended. In the middle of my second year, a third resident joined the clinic to provide a backup and potential replacement doctor. Approximately 80 percent of the women's fees were covered by Medicaid, other state-supported funding, or a sliding fee scale based on income.

This clinic, like most, was short of work space; examining rooms were the only place for doctors and staff to talk privately with individuals. All of the doctor-patient interactions took place in these rooms, with an occa-sional fleeting last-minute instruction or lab result being given the patient by the doctor in the hallways. Time was at a premium here with two people scheduled to see a doctor every fifteen minutes, and, once the clinic opened, the rush was on, from the crowded waiting room, to the bustle in the halls and triage space, to the filled examining rooms, to the hums and whirs in the lab. The director of the women's clinic, a women's health spe-cialist, did an exceptional job of juggling the staff, working to protect people's privacy while maintaining a smooth flow. The best plans, how-ever, tended to go awry. On a daily basis she often could not predict how many women needed to see a doctor, how many had more complicated problems than the staff had anticipated, how many would not show up or showed up late, how many unscheduled, desperate people did show up that the clinic felt it could not turn away, and so forth. Thus the clinic planned schedules, set up timetables, and hired staff knowing that at each session there would be a certain amount of mayhem.

Entering the second setting, the office of a well-established gynecologist in private practice, was a very different experience. Rather than stumbling over people, toys, and torn magazines in the waiting room, I felt as though I were walking into a well-appointed living room, with soft colors and textures and current glossy magazines. People arrived on time for appointments for which they did not have a long wait. Adamant that a full waiting room meant poor scheduling, this doctor insisted on short waits for his patients.

Medical encounters in the clinic were conducted in small examining rooms, but in this setting the examining rooms were larger and the doctor talked with people about outcomes and diagnoses in his office. The office was spacious with a large executive desk and leather-upholstered armchair for the doctor and matching chairs facing the desk for patients. The room was full of patients' charts and books. There was a statue of a mother and child. The walls were covered with awards, diplomas, and membership certificates. In sum, it was a comfortable room infused with the air that one would have a professional encounter with a very professional doctor who had special training in women's reproductive processes.

I began my fieldwork in the clinic, spending one year as a volunteer, observing all of the interactions, taking notes, and talking informally with patients and staff. In the second year I entered the private doctor's office while still observing in the clinic. During this second year I audiotaped doctor-patient interactions as I observed and conducted in-depth interviews with women in their homes. It was helpful to me as a researcher to be able simply to observe as a member of the group in the clinic for the first year, with permission by the director. By the time I began taping, I was an accepted presence in the setting and in a position to see to what degree the tape recorder changed the interactions. Any recording technology will introduce changes in interaction, but the impact seemed slight. In the clinic patients were used to a volunteer being present during exams, and thus my being there was not new. Women gave their permission to be taped, and the tape recorder was small and unobtrusive. In the beginning of the interaction some women seemed a little nervous, but it was difficult to tell whether this nervousness was because they were being recorded or because of the medical encounter. As the interaction went on, they seemed to forget about the recorder. When I asked women their impressions of being taped, many said they forgot about it once they became involved with the doctor. Others said they were aware of it but it did not bother them. All participants were told in advance that they could terminate their participation in the study at any time; none did. The doctors were all used to working in teaching hospitals, where examining rooms are often filled with observers and increasingly are videotaped for teaching material. Thus though the tape was an extra device, my impressions as well as those of the staff and patients were that it had minimum effect on their interactions.

It was much the same in the private practitioner's office. Here women were also used to observers in the examining rooms—medical students working with this doctor, the nurse, and so forth. Similarly, I noticed little difference between women's behavior before and after the tape was introduced. I did notice that when I first started observing, the doctor was somewhat stiff. I was not sure if this was his usual style or if my presence was affecting him. When I asked his nurse, she said he was "on his best behavior." I decided it was better not to tape until he became more used to me. After several weeks he seemed more relaxed, treating me as he did the rest of his staff—as a regular fixture. Once again, his nurse was an invaluable source of information. When I had been working there for a month she told me he was back to normal, whereupon I began the taping process.

In both settings I observed doctors in all of their activities. When I taped, however, I focused on women who had come in for birth control–related consultations. I hoped to observe the context in which well women were treated by doctors in settings that were organized around a disease model of delivery. Although some of the patients did fit this category, others combined a need for birth control–related information with a health problem. The reasons for this unexpected (for me) result were (1) that women often waited until they had several medical needs before seeking care, and (2) that the inducement of health problems by popular birth control methods often brings women to the doctor for more complicated care than I had anticipated.

The data base for this and the next chapter includes the observational data covering these two and one-half years and the detailed sociolinguistic analysis of twenty tapes, ten from each setting. To sociolinguists used to small segments of conversation or a case study, this body of data might seem large. To quantitative sociologists used to large panoramas of the population or demographic data, it might seem small. This "slice of life" is not meant to prove universal truths about health care delivery. Statistical significance is neither provided nor sought. Nor can it provide the linguistic detail found in analyses of small, single case study segments of conversation. Instead, it is my intention that the following detailed analysis be used against the backdrop of my observational notes and the research discussed in earlier chapters for better understanding of a subject in need of clarity—the doctor-patient relationship.

I will examine the organization of the doctor-patient interviews in three ways. First, distributional analysis is used to present an overview of all of the interactions. The conversations are broken down into types of speech used by doctors and patients. Second, the talk between participants is looked at in sequences. Turn-taking analysis used in combination with the distribution of speech patterns gives us a broader view of the form of the data. And third, the content of the conversations is explored to learn what topics doctors and women discuss.

DISTRIBUTIONAL ANALYSIS

In recent years observers from many disciplines have had much to say about our medical system, but actual interactions between medical staff and patients have received less attention. Sociologists have traditionally viewed language as a static phenomenon. Nevertheless, though it is as invisible as the air we breathe, it is just as important. Interactional encounters both reflect and maintain the more abstract arrangements of society. It is with a commitment to a conception of language as an active force in the understanding of social life that I will discuss conversations between gynecologists and patients from both of the medical settings described above.

Medical encounters—often criticized for being too brief—result in substantial transcripts when taped. What seems like a short conversation can become pages of utterances that, once transcribed with all the "ums," "ahs," start overs, and interruptions, take on a new and lengthy complexity. By breaking up doctors' and patients' discourse into types of speech, it is possible to begin to see the structure of who is saying what to whom, who is doing most of the talking, what forms this talk takes, and how it reflects and supports the distribution of power in the medical relationship.

Speech act theory provides a useful springboard for analyzing the quantities of data that result from taping conversations. This theory, as outlined by J. L. Austin (1962) and John Searle (1969)[2] and influenced by the writings of Ludwig Wittgenstein, treats speech as a social activity based on the intentions of everyday people using what is called "natural language." Conversations are broken up into units of speech based on their intended action—questions, statements, and so forth. The basic unit of research has been defined as the sentence, broken into these patterns of use. Roy D'Andrade (n.d.) suggests that to analyze actual conversations between people, six categories of speech acts are needed: statements, questions, expressives, directives, reactives, and commissives (see Table 1).

TABLE 1.
D'Andrade's Preliminary Speech Act Category System

A. *Statements* (expositives, representatives, assertions)
  Reports
  Quotes
  Instantiations
  Claims
  Stimulations (?)
  Inferences
B. *Directives* (requests, orders, exercitives)
  Suggest/request/order
  Request object
  Agree as to truth
  Expression of approval, sympathy, support
  Commitment
  Direct action
  Direct/indirect
C. *Questions*
  Wh-form
  Yes-no form
  Tag form
  Intonation only form
  Information only versus other uses

D. *Reactives* (agreement or disagreement with what has previously been stated)
  Agree as to truth versus disagree as to truth
  Give attention
  Accede (agree to commit or actually do) versus refuse
E. *Expressives*
  Give approval versus disapproval
  Sympathy, regret, exasperation
  Direct versus indirect (accusation, disagreements)
F. *Commissives*
  Promise, offer, vow

I have adapted these categories for my own use, abridging the system in the process to fit the specific requirements for tabulating speech acts in the medical interview. My revisions exclude expressives and commissives. Although these actions take place in the medical setting, they do so subtly and in the form of statements, questions, and directives. Strong emotion is not considered appropriate in the gynecologist-patient relationship, and actions such as vowing or showing exasperation tend to be played down and absorbed into other acts. I have subdivided reactives into two categories—reactives and answers. Speech acts will be considered answers when they provide a substantive response to a question. They will be considered reactives when used to acknowledge a statement, as shown in the following example from a clinic tape.

1. Doctor: You've just finished your period?

2. Patient: Uh hum.

3. Doctor: Okay.

As this excerpt shows, the doctor first makes a statement that has the effect of eliciting information from a woman patient. I have coded the doctor's sentence (1) as a question because of its interrogative tone and because the doctor receives an answer (2). The doctor then acknowledges the patient's answer with a reactive (3). I have determined the meaning of these conversational acts on the basis of their *function* in speech rather than their inherent grammatical form. The classification system used for my data thus consists of statements (S), questions (Q), reactives (R), answers (A), and directives (D) applied to conversations between the doctor (D) and the patient (P).

In Table 2 the data have been separated and tabulated into speech acts of doctors and patients in the twenty taped interactions. These interactions were conversations centered on some aspect of contraceptive care. Analysis of discourse showed both similarities and differences between medical care in the two settings studied. First the similarities:

1. The doctors asked more questions than did the patients. In the clinic the doctors asked 5.6 times as many questions as the patients. The private practitioner asked 11.5 times as many questions as the patients.

2. As a logical consequence, patients provided more answers than doctors—in the clinic, 5.6 times more, in the private practice, 19 times.

3. The doctors made more statements than the patients—about twice as many in both settings.

4. Doctors (with one exception) made all the directives.

There were also differences:

1. The gap between questions asked by the doctors and questions asked by the patients was greater in the private practitioner's office than in the clinic. Doctors and patients in the clinic asked more questions, but patients in the private practitioner's office asked very few questions.

2. The same was true of answers to these questions. The patients in the private doctor's office not only asked fewer questions but received fewer answers. Further, the patients in this office received fewer answers to questions asked than did the patients in the clinic.

3. In the clinic the doctors uttered more reactives than the patients. The reverse was true in the private office.

4. Directives were used less frequently by the clinic doctors than the private practitioner.

These findings give us useful information about who says what to whom and how (see Hymes 1972). The tabulation of speech acts provides an overview of the data in the form of a distributional analysis which divides talk into discrete components, showing the similarities and differences in the structure of the conversations in the two settings investi-

TABLE 2.
Aggregate of Speech Acts

Speech Acts	Statements D	P	Questions D	P	Answers D	P	Reactives D	P	Directives D	P	Subtotals D	P	Totals
Clinic													
Number	210	92	251	45	42	244	220	123	69	–	792	504	1,296
Percent	70	30	85	15	15	85	64	36	100	–	61	39	100
Dr. M													
Number	248	122	185	16	9	167	139	225	158	1	739	531	1,270
Percent	67	33	92	8	5	95	38	62	99	1	58	42	100

This distribution is based on the discourse between doctor and patient in the examination room in the clinic and the examination and office consultation in Dr. M's office.

Key: D = doctor; P = patient.

gated (see Frankel 1983 and West 1984 for their discussion of questions in doctor-patient communication). Comparisons suggest a preliminary view of the distribution of talk and power in the medical interview. We see the doctor doing much of the talking and using the more active, initiating types of speech in both settings.

The tabulation of speech acts is informative. It is also important to understand its limitations. Speech act theory provides a skeleton upon which to hang further analyses. For though this dissection provides speech tabulated into active parts, it does not offer information about the way the doctors and women act in concert, influencing each other in the course of the interaction—it lacks the interconnectedness of the encounter. A sequential relationship of who asks or states what speech act when and how these utterances are ordered between the two can offer the beginnings of a broader view from which to understand doctor-patient communication.

SEQUENTIAL ORDER

The doctor-patient discourse takes place in the institutional setting of health care delivery. In this system doctors have power as experts and often as males. Women participate in an exchange of information which is structured by who does the talking and who dominates the turns of talk. The institutional setting influences this sequencing, constraining the form of the interaction. The discourse and the organization reflect and sustain each other to produce the health care delivered.

To make this point clearer it is helpful to compare the structure of language used in everyday interactions with that used in institutions such as medicine, where the discussion is more specific and tends to take on certain patterns.[3] Conversation analysts have revealed a two-part structure in conversation between equal participants in everyday settings. One person asks a question, the other person answers; or one person makes a statement and the other comments, the turns continuing in this fashion (this is an ideal type, not necessarily the format of all conversations). Researchers have found that the dialogue between individuals is organized differently in some institutions. The difference seems to be a consequence of the asymmetry between participants, which produces a third part to the conversation (see Fisher [1986] for her analysis of comment acts and third pair parts in the medical interview; see West [1984] for her detailed discussion of how turn-taking analysis can be used to improve doctor-patient communication). In the educational setting this third part is an evaluation act: the teacher evaluates the work that the students are doing— the teacher asks a question, a student answers, and the teacher evaluates the response, thus bringing control of the floor back to the teacher to ask the next question (Mehan 1979).

In the medical data analyzed here, the third part of the conversational sequences is a reactive; it is used by the doctor to maintain control of the floor. The doctor initiates a request for information, receives information from the patient, and acknowledges the answer with a reactive. The doctor's reactive serves two purposes: (1) the doctor initiates the interaction with a question, and in so doing determines the topic or the direction of the conversation; (2) after the patient responds, the doctor (like the teacher) uses the reactive (evaluation) to maintain control of the floor, introducing a new topic or continuing on in the sequence already started.

Initiation	*Reply*	*Acknowledgment*
D:Q	*P:A*	*D:R*
So you haven't had a period since then?	No.	All right.

In this sequence the doctor's "all right" acknowledges the woman's reply and sets the doctor up to continue.

D:S	*P:R*	*D:R*
Chances are if you're not having your		
period, you're not ovulating.	Um hum.	Okay.

My data indicate that the doctors initiate the sequences and topics introducing speech acts which effectively shape the content and direction of the encounter. The patients' conversations also contain reactives, but there is a difference. The patients' reactives differ from those of the doctor in that they occur as single speech act turns. The women do not generally utter a reactive and then continue with this same turn. Rather, they use the reactive as a courtesy or acknowledgment to indicate that they understand or are listening, adding nothing more.

My findings concerning the use of reactives in the two medical settings indicate some subtle and some not so subtle organizational and interactional influences on discourse. In both settings, the doctors' conversations exhibit how reactives provide the means for changing topics, effectively maintaining control over the conversation; the doctors thereby exhibit medical-institutional power through speech exchange. Much of the research discussed in earlier chapters highlights doctors' ability to wield this control. In this chapter discourse analysis shows how they do so. These patterns were discernible in both settings, with the doctors having more control over the talk than the patients. Exactly how this was accomplished, however, was different. The private practitioner (Dr. M) used fewer reactives than the clinic doctors and the women seeing him used more. The private practitioner also used more directives than did clinic doctors. Dr. M used directives to change topics, often doing so abruptly, talking over the women. Thus though clinic doctors primarily used reactives to change topics, Dr. M used both reactives and directives for that purpose. He also used directives at a far higher rate than did the clinic doctors in instructing women about treatment decisions.

The following examples involve two women, one from each setting, who came to the doctor for treatment of amenorrhea (cessation of menstruation). Both also sought renewal of birth control pill prescriptions. The woman coming to the clinic wanted to resume use of the pill after a lapse of several months. The woman seeing Dr. M came for a routine renewal of her prescription. Analysis of the transcripts displays the very different styles of the two doctors. This difference is observable in comparisons of the tapes from the two settings even when the transcripts are of the other clinic doctors. Such comparisons suggest that the difference lies in the organizational arrangements, not simply in individual styles. In the clinic, the doctor attempts to explain the problem to the woman, using statements as the major form of imparting instructions and information. Dr. M uses directives to a far greater degree, both to mention new aspects of a problem and to impart instructions.

EXAMPLE 1

Clinic doctor	*Patient*
(S) I discussed your problem with one of the head doctors at General, uhm, he knows more about this than I do, about amenorrhea, not getting your period, and he seemed to think, uhm, he seemed to agree with me that it would probably be a good idea to give a test dose of this progesterone to see if you have a withdrawal bleeding. I assume that this is probably what you were injected with earlier this summer, that was the injection, progesterone, that's a hormone in your body that makes your uterus shed its lining and you bleed, okay, and it works, progesterone is a normal hormone that works in regular cycles. Now, uhm, since you don't have any strong desires to get pregnant at this point, since you did come here for/ contraception, uhm, we both seem to think that it would be, uhm, the best idea to give you the progesterone for five days, have	(R) /Right.

a withdrawal bleed, and then start
you on the pill.
(Q) Okay?   (R) Okay.
(S) (D) And if you don't get a
withdrawal bleed with progesterone,
it's a pill which you'll take for
five days, if you don't, call us
and then we'll see you and we'll
have to give you—well have to go
through another test before we start
you on something.
(Q) Okay?
(S) Now, uhm, just judging from what,
you know, from your story, you
told me that you did have a little
spotting/   (R) /Uh hum.
from the injection, it sounds
like you, you just haven't been
ovulating so this could be a
problem when you do try to get
pregnant, you know, when you do
want to get pregnant again, we'll
have to get you on regular cycles
where you're ovulating in order
for you to get pregnant.
(Q) Okay?   (Q) Now, this
                                                    time if I take it
                                                    for five days,
                                                    what happens
                                                    if I just start
                                                    bleeding?

(A) That's—even the slightest amount
is okay.
(Q) Okay?
(S) Even if it's just a little spot.
It doesn't have to be like a real
period, just, you know, a little
spot here and there. You might
want to wear a mini pad or something.   (R) Okay.

EXAMPLE 2

Private Practitioner   *Patient*
   EXAM:
   (D) Look,
(S) what I think is happening, that your
pills are not strong enough,
(Q) you know?
(S) I've put you on a very low pill as you

know/   (R) /Right.
and sometimes this will cause
(swallows word). Now what I would like
to do is when you finish your pills.
Let's see, you're on the twenty-eight days.
(long pause)   (R) Right. (S)
                                     Uh, twenty-one
                                     day.

(R) Twenty-one day, all right.
(D) When you finish your pills, and if
you don't menstruate within five to six
days, come in.
(S) I won't charge you anything if I don't
have to do anything and I will give
you a prescription for a different
kind. I want to see what you're going
to do. I also want you to report back
on this.   (R) Right,
                                     uh hum.
(Q) Okay?   (R) Oh, okay.

     CONSULTATION:
     (D) Now, look,
(S) what I want to do, you understand now,
all right, you have X number of tablets,
(D) then you finish the package,
(Q) Right?   (R) Right.
(R) Right.
(D) Finish them wait four to five days.
If you flow, come in then while you're
flowing and I'll, uh, uh, and I'll give
you more pills. (long pause)   (R) Okay.
(S) I won't charge you.
(D) If you don't flow, call me,
(S) then I will give you an injection,
(D) don't take any more tablets then.   (R) Uh hum.
(S) I'll give you an injection and I'll,
un, get you started with your
menstruation and I'll give you a
different type of pill. (long pause)   (R) Okay.
(Q) Okay?   (R) All right.
(D) But meanwhile, stay on the pills.
(D) Don't you get into trouble.   (R) Right.

Examples 1 and 2 indicate that Dr. M's directives such as "Finish them wait four or five days" provide him with control of the floor much as the reactives "okay" and "all right" provided control for the clinic doctors. The doctor in each setting did most of the talking about the women's concerns (as shown in Table 2). The doctors uttered multiple speech acts per turn in both examples—making statements, asking questions—and the women answered questions or acknowledged information in single or double speech act turns. The distribution of questions and answers in the doctor-patient interviews in both settings shows the doctor asking more questions and the patient providing more answers. In addition, Dr. M more often solicited a response from women. The clinic doctors tagged questions such as "Okay?" onto their directions, or gave expectant looks to women seeking confirmation of understanding, but they never, in my observations, insisted on a response. In fact, they so often rushed through such solicitations in their talk that the patient was scarcely able, let alone required, to respond. Dr. M, however, used tag questions, "Okay?" "Right?" or long pauses accompanied by a piercing, direct gaze to accomplish acknowledgment, in some cases repeating this procedure for emphasis. In Example 2, Dr. M states, "I also want you to report back on this," emphasizing the words with direct eye contact. The patient responds with a double reactive, "Right, uh hum," to reassure him that she will do her part. Dr. M responds with a tag question, "Okay?" for further emphasis, eliciting acknowledgment again from this woman in the form of another reactive, "Oh, okay."

The similarities in speech composition in the settings as exemplified in the above two examples can be explained by the fact that all of the doctors have been trained in the same biomedical model and hold the same basic assumptions on how health care should be delivered. There are, however, differences, which can be attributed in part to the organizational arrangements of the two settings. Dr. M, a private practitioner, sitting behind his big desk, his nurse bringing him coffee, fetching him charts, and ushering in women, exerts a great deal of power in his interactions with *his* patients. Little happens in this office that Dr. M does not know about, organize, and control. Women interact solely with Dr. M concerning their reasons for visiting a doctor. Their power lies in choosing or choosing not to come to this doctor, challenging the doctor face-to-face (which I never saw happen), not returning, or complying with or ignoring the doctor's instructions. In my observations, when women were dissatisfied, the strongest reaction against Dr. M in the interaction was silence, or an attempt at silence, as in the following excerpt—the most extreme in my data taken from field notes:

> The doctor turned his attention to the patient and started examining her breasts, which were quite large. As he was looking at her breasts, she was flat on her back staring at the ceiling. Dr. M said, "Yes, this is all girl," and smiled at the patient. No one in the room—the patient, the medical assistant, or myself—acknowledged the doctor's remark. The room was unusually quiet as the doctor started checking the patient's other breast. He slowly and measuredly

started talking while looking around at each one of us, "I *said*, this is all girl." At this point the patient smiled wanly, the medical assistant chuckled, and I smiled. With our responses the doctor's good humor returned and he told the patient to "get dressed like a good girl" and he would give her "some more happy pills" [birth control pills].

In this interaction Dr. M exerted power in two ways. First, he made a statement, which, in the absence of a response, he reiterated. Although speakers have rights to reassert that which is not responded to, it seems clear that the lack of response was deliberate, rather than not having been heard or understood. That the doctor demanded and received acquiescence from everyone present regarding a topic independent of the woman's health needs constitutes a form of power. Second, while performing the breast exam the physician reinforced gender-based stereotypes of female anatomy in a way that seems incongruous with the purpose of screening for cancer.[4]

The clinic doctors, in contrast, displayed no possessiveness toward the patients. They did control the floor and dominate the interaction with much the same outcome as in Dr. M's office, but the process had a different feel. Women in the clinic were seen by rotating doctors in an atmosphere where it is acknowledged that women have other informational resources such as volunteers and so forth. Whereas Dr. M exercised sole control, the clinic doctor was only one possible step in several. Interestingly, women seeing Dr. M asked fewer questions than did women in the clinic; it is possible that they felt less active and more dominated or intimidated in Dr. M's office.[5]

The structure of the conversations that I have recorded between doctors and women can be seen to reflect the institutional power of medicine. Having determined this structure, the next step in understanding the broader picture is to examine what is said—the content of the conversations. The content of these discussions illuminates medical dominance even more clearly, showing how it shapes *what* is talked about as well as *how* the conversation is linguistically organized.

CONTENT ANALYSIS

The sequential analysis of the doctor-patient interview provides a framework for building on speech act distribution. The more abstract institutional and organizational arrangements of the medical profession can be seen in the daily interactions between doctors and women. Examination of the interconnections between the level of discourse and the level of institutionally designated power offers useful information for further study of the doctor-patient relationship and health care delivery.

In conversations that take place in everyday life and in institutional situations, information is arranged by topic. Neither the distributional nor the sequential properties reveal the content of the medical interview. When the data are examined with the content as the focus, the uniqueness of the doctor–female patient relationship begins to emerge.

Several patterns are of relevance in the data I collected. First, doctors' interpretations took precedence over women's understandings. For example, in the following excerpt from the clinic, a woman complains of dizziness, bloating, tiredness, and general dissatisfaction that she feels is caused by a five-year course of birth control pills. The doctor is skeptical that the birth control pill is the cause of these problems.

EXAMPLE 3

Doctor

Do, do your legs swell, is that part of your problem or do you just feel kinda bloated?

/Uh hum. Sometimes things get blamed on the pills that aren't always the pills' fault so, like/

women who say they gained weight because they're taking the pills when ordinarily they're expecting to gain weight, so maybe they eat a little bit more, and, uh, then they gain weight and say, oh, look at the pill made me gain weight.

I've never heard that one before (laughs).

Patient

My, I don't know my stomach just feels really, like it's out here, you know, very/

/What?

But it makes me hungry. When I'm not on the pill, I don't feel hungry.

The doctor laughs off the woman's concerns about the birth control pill. She, however, is worried about the relationship between her health and contraceptive method. Her worries go unaddressed by a doctor who dismisses her interpretation of the problem. But her concerns are neither surprising nor unreasonable. All of her symptoms are known effects of the pill, discussed by researchers, doctors, congressional hearings, the popular press, and women's health groups. The birth control pill may be useful to this woman, depending on her need to avoid pregnancy, but the concerns she expressed are legitimate and deserve careful consideration—a consideration she did not receive.

In the following example of interpretational dominance, Dr. M and a woman who has come to him for several years discuss medical insurance.

EXAMPLE 4

Doctor	Patient
Uh, Nancy, anything you need, you know that from previous times, you just see me, you know, anything medical, you know. And what I would suggest, now you have a choice between Kaiser [an HMO] and Blue Cross, I think (pause)—take	
	Uh hum.
Blue Cross. You don't need anything for office calls. You're not going to go broke on that; you know that (pause).	
	Uh hum.
Uh, but you should have some hospital and surgery, so if you want to stay with me, you know, and, uh, I would suggest that you just take Blue Cross on the hospital and surgical, you know, uh, then you can come to me.	
	Okay.
You know, since you feel that strongly about it, you know.	
	But does Blue Cross cover like examinations when you have a physical?
Honey, this is what I'm trying to tell you. Look, yes.	
	I don't think they do.
Some do, some don't. But that basically is not what you need. Now you're not going to go broke by coming once or twice a year for a pelvic examination.	
	Yeah.

While Nancy tried to assert her concerns, the doctor, increasingly impatient, insisted that he knew what she needed, and it was obvious to him what she should do. It was not so obvious to Nancy. But in the end, both of the above women accepted the view that "the doctor knows best." The former left with her birth control prescription feeling that if she could only diet and eat properly, her problems with the pill would disappear. The latter decided on Blue Cross insurance despite her continued worries about the probable extra expense of doctor visits not covered by this plan.[6]

A second impression from the observations is that the doctors' more dominant reasoning often led to condescension, which was observable in sequences throughout the interviews in both settings. The doctors in the clinic were more likely than Dr. M to explain to a woman what they were doing, but still they often seemed to be talking down to her, as if to a child. The exchange in Example 5 represents a pattern common in the clinic when women observed their cervix by using a mirror during the exam.

EXAMPLE 5

Doctor	Patient
You can hold the mirror and you can just kind of angle it in and see it [cervix]. Can you see it?	Oh, yeah.
It's like a little pink doughnut?	Uh huh.
It's got a little hole.	Uh huh.
That's where the baby comes out.	

The doctors used the diminutive "little" in many of their explanations—in such statements as the one in the above example; in initiating an exam ("I'm just going to do a little exam"); in applying medication to vaginal warts ("a little bit on that one and a little bit on this one"); and in teaching women breast self-examination ("just march your little fingers"). Further, this is an example of how, when explaining a woman's anatomy to her, the clinic doctors' descriptions were tied not to the cervix as a part of her body, but rather to the role it played in having babies, whether or not she had expressed an interest in reproducing.

Dr. M always examined women in the more conventional manner, without explaining his actions. But he often showed a condescending attitude toward patients in his belief, expressed to me and to them, that they would not comply with his advice. He did not explore this alleged lack of compliance to discover its roots, but rather assumed that women were unreliable and needed constant admonishing about their health care. In statements to a Mexican-American woman regarding her use of birth control, he asserted, "Okay. I've given it to you in English and Spanish. Now you better mind it, okay?" In the following example, Dr. M addresses a woman who has run out of birth control pills and must wait until her next cycle to resume taking them.

EXAMPLE 6

Doctor	Patient
Okay, now, honey, look, so that you don't get pregnant again, I want you to	

get this foam, okay?   Uh hum.
You go to the drugstore and get it, and
then here are the instructions. Read it.
Now it's very simple.
[This woman had not been pregnant recently.]

Dr. M's "honey" and the step-by-step instructions were typically uttered slowly and carefully, as if to a small child. He often included favorite expressions such as "Have you been a good girl?" meaning "Have you used contraception responsibly?" and "Here are your happy pills" meaning birth control pills. These phrases usually elicited nervous laughs and twitches from women.

A third finding suggested by my data is one I talk about in much greater detail in the next chapter: doctors and women framed their conversations in very different ways—the former predominantly in medical, general terms, with some social talk, and the latter in more social, biographical styles with some medical talk. These categories are ideal types that represent dichotomies assumed in the medical model and Western culture in general. They are not, however, so clearly demarcated in actual practice. It is thus useful to think of them as placed along a continuum from the contextual to the biomedical, knowing that each end has shades of the other extreme (see Mishler 1984, Silverman and Torode 1980). The doctor-patient interviews that I observed and taped present primarily biomedical conversations centered around a physiologically treated and defined issue—for example, the need to renew a prescription or amenorrhea and its possible connections to use of the birth control pill—with contextual nuances inserted here and there.

Birth control, however, has more than technical significance for women (Luker 1975, Todd 1983). The choice and use of contraceptives interrelate with sexual relationships, contextual circumstances, and life choices. Whereas the doctor speaks from a technical, biological standpoint, the patient's speech is often social and contextual.[7] As I noted earlier, doctors exert more control in the interaction than do patients, so that the exchange of information is primarily technical in nature. When patients do take control of the floor, their topics center on the wider social context of their health and their bodies, as seen in Example 7.

EXAMPLE 7

Doctor   *Patient*
                                            Uh, I haven't
                                            been here lately
                                            because I had to
                                            switch to Kaiser

for financial rea-
sons and I've
been on a leave
of absence and
they can't take
me back for a
while.

Uh huh. What pills are you on now?

This woman has visited the clinic for birth control pill renewal and has introduced several topics: (1) failure to visit the clinic; (2) an alternative health plan; (3) financial matters; (4) leave of absence from her job; and (5) loss of work. The doctor provides a token acknowledgment of her comments, immediately changing the topic to the birth control pill. The conversation in this example fails to strike a balance between the topics of concern to the woman and the doctor's narrower, biomedical focus. The patient is talking in a social, contextual mode about her health care and her life. The doctor responds with a medical, prescription-oriented question, taking the conversation back into the medical domain. This person considers her understandings of her life circumstances relevant to her health care; financial matters and the change of medical facilities, combined with a leave of absence and loss of work, are important concerns potentially affecting her health and care. Since he does not probe, the doctor leaves her concerns unacknowledged, tinged with an air of the inappropriate, a situation that effectively disregards her topics.

The interchange in Example 8 takes place during a routine pelvic exam and gynecological checkup for renewal of a prescription for birth control pills.

EXAMPLE 8

Doctor

Okay, I'm going to take a little bit of your secretion to look at it to make sure you don't have an infection, too. Okay, coming out, you're doing fine. Stay right there now. Doing all right Norma?

Patient

I feel uneasy tonight, I don't know why.

Well, we're almost done. Relax. Okay, your cervix's right there. Right behind your bladder.

This woman has reported a vaginal discharge. Throughout the interaction she has appeared depressed and has expressed dissatisfaction with her birth control method. In this brief excerpt she tentatively makes a so-

TABLE 3.
Aggregate of Speech Acts Divided into Medical and Social Content

Speech Acts	Statements D	P	Questions D	P	Answers D	P	Reactives D	P	Directives D	P	Subtotals D	P	Totals
Clinic													
Dominant style													
Medical	181	62	229	39	35	214	204	108	67	–	716	423	1,139
Social	29	30	22	6	7	30	16	15	2	–	76	81	157
Percentage of speech acts													
Medical	16	5	20	3	3	19	18	10	6	–	63	37	100
Social	19	19	14	4	4	19	10	10	1	–	48	52	100
Dr. M													
Dominant style													
Medical	197	67	141	12	5	126	119	194	146	1	608	400	1,008
Social	51	55	44	4	4	41	20	31	12	–	131	131	262
Percentage of speech acts													
Medical	19	7	14	1	1	13	12	19	14	–	60	40	100
Social	19	21	17	2	2	16	7	12	4	–	49	51	100

cial statement about her mood. The doctor's response incorporates this comment into a technical explanation relating to the exam and directs her to relax, changing the topic back to the physiological.

The above examples highlight patterns of women's social, contextual topics related to their health. Doctors also engage in social talk when treating patients. The insertion of such topics into the medical discourse occurs frequently enough in the data to require explanation and infrequently enough to constitute a breach or break in the typical interactional flow. Table 3 shows that although social talk represents a small percentage of the conversation, it does occur. Once again, a more detailed analysis is needed to see the similarities and the differences in the ways patients and doctors use social topics.

Some social conversations centered around an exchange between doctors and women based on shared contextual knowledge. For example, a clinic doctor commented on a woman's New England accent, triggering a discussion of the doctor's medical school years in Massachusetts. In Dr. M's office, the social talk was an equal exchange of information regarding a woman's trip or similar pleasantries. For the most part, however, social comments were isolated remarks embedded in or eliciting a change back to a medical, technical format. Sequences in the discourse show a weaving back and forth between social and medical topics, with social topics in the minority.

The discourse also shows a difference in ways the doctors and the women talk about social issues. Usually women's mentions of social issues were particularistic and contextual, relating to their lives in ways they considered pertinent to the discussion of their bodies. In Example 9, for instance, the doctor presents general medical knowledge to explain why menstrual periods temporarily cease after a woman stops taking the pill.

EXAMPLE 9

Doctor	Patient
Okay, push back and sit up. Sometimes after you go off the pill, you cannot have your period for a while and that's not abnormal, to not have a period.	
	Uhh, before I had my daughter, my husband was stationed, or no, it was after I had Sally, he was stationed overseas and I went off the pill

and my period
started like six
weeks after.

The woman responds with a particularistic, social statement weaving her own body's cycles with contextual, family information. The sequence in Example 10 shows a similar medical-social distinction between the doctor's question and the woman's answer; Example 11 exhibits the woman's contextual understanding of her body and reproduction during a visit to her doctor's office.

EXAMPLE 10

Doctor	Patient
Yeah. When was the last time that it did something like this, was late [menstruation].	I missed one once right before my wedding. That was in September, but that was because I was so nervous, I mean we were moving all around so/

EXAMPLE 11

Doctor	Patient
Your pregnancy test is negative. That makes us happy.	Okay, doctor. It makes me happy, especially since I broke up with him three months ago.

Doctors also made social comments regarding women's reproductive circumstances, but they differed in that these comments reflected general, stereotypic attitudes. The doctors voiced an abstract, social understanding, often of women's traditional roles, triggered by the specific situation of the topic being discussed. The sequence presented in Example 12 follows Dr. M's direction not to have intercourse for two or three weeks because this woman has a new baby.

EXAMPLE 12

Doctor	Patient
	Don't worry. I keep telling you people I could take it or leave it, preferably leave it.
Look, honey, you have a husband don't you.	
	Yeah, I know (resignedly).

This woman expressed her disinclination for sexual activity at the present, and Dr. M volunteered a stereotypic comment on women's responsibilities as sexual partners in marriage. He did not probe for information about her current sexual disinterest or initiate discussion of ways for her to understand her present situation. In the following example, Dr. M, in lecturing to a woman on taking her birth control pills properly and the risks of missing them, exhibited similar traditional attitudes toward marriage and pregnancy.

EXAMPLE 13

Doctor	Patient
Now why did you stop [the pill]?	I don't know. They kept telling me it's bad. . . .
Now who are you going to listen to? People or your doctor? . . . You know, and you're going to, uh, particularly since you're not married, you're going to take care of it [baby] and you're going to have all the problems. . . .	
	(nods head)
You start the pills, you know, and come in. I'll write you another prescription for more pills.	

Dr. M here displays the cultural assumption that marriage comes before pregnancy and draws on it when he urges this woman to use birth control properly. He is inserting his own conventional wisdom into a conversation in which the woman's social talk is discouraged.

Similar conventional views of women's roles can be seen in the clinic interaction in Example 14. The doctor discourages a woman from an intrauterine device (IUD) for several good reasons, including the possibility that she would jeopardize her future fertility and the possibility of death, and encourages her to use the birth control pill. (All of the doctors observed in my study generally opposed the IUD, preferring the birth control pill.) As the italicized lines indicate, however, counseling on women's roles is interwoven with medical advice.

EXAMPLE 14

Doctor

I, I have a very negative opinion of the IUD, *particularly for young women who haven't had their family yet,* because if/

Patient

/Uhm, they give it to girls who have abortions and miscarriages. Why, why is that?

I think that's just because it's, the, the women don't feel that they could take the pill, and it's some, it's some form of birth control, at least. For women who just can't remember to take the pill or won't, that need protection, then the IUD is some (pause), you know, is second best. But you're really taking a big chance of infection. We're seeing at least I'd say five in a hundred IUDs that we put in are coming back with some, some sort of infection, often not serious, but it can be very serious. It can mean hospitalization and antibiotics into your veins, and some of them even have their organs operated on or removed because they get so infected, it can even result in death, then, you know, so it's, again, a remote possibility the same as blood clots are with the birth control pills, although it's not as remote as that. It happens, it really, you know, much more frequently. *Uhm, I think the scariest thing, even if, you know, you don't get overwhelming infection, with the IUD is that we don't know what we, what your future fertility would be like.* The IUD works by causing a little infection inside your

uterus and it can climb up inside the
tubes and it may destroy the normal
structure of the tubes enough so that
the egg, which is very small, and the
tube, which is also very small, don't fit,
and they can get hung up. There's a/ /I see.
higher incidence of ectopic pregnancy,
tubal pregnancies, when the egg stops
in the tube and then tries to grow into
a baby there, with women who've had IUDs. Oh, I see.
So I, I really think, unless you're really
adamant and you, you're willing to take
all those chances, I really wouldn't tend,
wouldn't recommend it. (laugh) Okay,
that answers/
/So it sounds like maybe the pill really
is the right thing.

(Note: Emphasis added.)

The social assumptions of the doctor in this example center around
the future fertility of the young, single woman who seeks contraception. There is an assumption, first, that she will one day want children,
and second, that despite possible infection, surgery, and death, the IUD is
the contraceptive most to be feared as a potential cause of infertility. The
discussion implies that for a woman who already had a family, the potential dangers of infection, surgery, and death, although still problems,
would not be so serious. It is important that reproductive capacity as well
as life be preserved and not jeopardized by medical technology. The slant,
however, toward one form of contraception thought by some to be dangerous (the pill) and away from another also considered a risk (the IUD)
shows a social bias masked as objective fact.

Interestingly, this woman and doctor would contend that the woman
had chosen her birth control method herself. They are correct, but there
was considerable persuasion in the decision-making process (see Fisher
and Todd 1986).[8] Doctors from both settings assumed the role of protector
of the reproductive function as in the above example. They also discouraged reproductive carelessness (Example 15). In this form of social talk,
the doctors engaged in "keeping the moral order" (Fisher 1986). To a
white, middle-class, married woman, Dr. M said in a friendly, chatty manner, "Now look, Susan, uh, this is the third time [abortion]. I'm talking as
a friend to you as well as your doctor, okay?" In Example 15, however, the
doctor takes a different tone. This patient is a young black woman, single
and receiving Medicaid.

EXAMPLE 15

Doctor	Patient
Look, you already had two abortions,	
at seventeen.	I know this.
Well!?!	But the next
	time I become
	pregnant, I'm
	gonna keep it.
Yeah, but I mean at seventeen and	
being single, do you want to be	
pregnant?	

The doctor was far sterner in talking to her about her reproductive history and future than he had been with the married woman. Dr. M strongly disapproved of pregnancies among single women and in conversations with me referred to women in this group as "stupid" and "irresponsible." Whether teenage pregnancies, IUD use, and so forth are desirable or undesirable are not the issues here. Rather, under the guise of medical treatment, cultural values about women's proper behavior and roles are being asserted.

The private practitioner was confidently vocal in his views and advice—both technical and social—to women. The clinic doctors were rarely so explicit. One doctor, in treating a twenty-one-year-old single woman for postabortion pain, did not discuss her failure to use birth control until the end of the interaction. As he was concluding the exam and preparing to leave the room, he grimly directed her: "Okay, well, use your diaphragm. Use it every time, remember to take it out every time." Throughout the exam, this woman had expressed intense pain. The doctor had ignored her signals and moans. As the doctor and I left the examining room, he rolled his eyes at me and said, "She acts like she's fourteen years old." Both settings included such opinions; in the office of Dr. M, they formed part of the discourse between doctor and patient whereas in the clinic they tended to receive subtler expression in the examining room, being more openly voiced among staff members.

CONCLUSION

The research reviewed in Chapters 1 and 2 made clear that the doctor-patient relationship is a troubled one, especially when the patient is a woman. The analyses presented in this chapter provide some detail into the dynamics of these troubles. Patriarchal assumptions and hierarchical arrangements throughout American society are both reflected and reinforced in the institution of medicine. The intention here has been to take the reader into the examining room, to observe, firsthand, some connections among attitudes toward women, power relationships, and communication.

In this body of data, the distributional analysis suggests that doctors talked the most, directing the conversations. The sequential orderings show how the speech acts work in concert, how doctors orchestrate (for the most part unconsciously) control of the floor, and how they dominate the topics to be discussed. In the section above looking at the content of these conversations we can see how, although the biomedical is the most prevalent form of talk, the use of the social is important in the medical interview. Both doctors and patients expressed social attitudes and concerns. Doctors' general attitudes toward women and reproduction came out repeatedly. Women's more particularistic understandings, when raised (often tentatively), were usually discouraged or ignored by the doctors, who returned to biomedical topics. It is these later interactions, in particular, that most intrigue me. Why, for instance, does the doctor in Example 8 assume in a kindly way that the patient is uneasy about the pelvic exam and return the conversation to these procedures? This woman specifically stated that she was uneasy "tonight," a night, in fact, when she was considering a change of contraceptive method. Possible complexities surrounding this change are not pursued. In the next chapter the specific dynamics of what is talked about and, even more interesting, what is not talked about are explored in more depth.

NOTES

1. This chapter is a revision of my article "The Prescription of Contraception: Negotiations Between Doctors and Patients," *Discourse Processes* 7 (April–June, 1984): 171–200. The title of this chapter is in part taken from my article "'The Patient Doesn't Have Anything to Say about It': Communications Between Gynecologists and Women Patients," in *Gewalt Durch Sprache: Die Vergewaltigung von Frauen in Gesprachen,* ed. Senta Tromel-Plotz (Frankfurt: Fischer Taschenbuch Verlag, 1984). This and the following conversations are taken verbatim from my data base of audiotaped interviews between doctors and women. I was present during both interactions. The expanded explanations that accompany these examples are taken from my interviews with the women.

2. Noam Chomsky's (1968) view of linguistics addressed the relationship between linguistic form and meaning in syntactic terms, with the sentence as the unit of analysis—a long tradition of looking at "autonomous language." Searle (1969) differs from Chomsky by distinguishing between the propositional content of utterances and elocutionary force or intention to act on the world. This shifts the focus from the linguistic emphasis on syntax to an analysis of function and the relationship between language and action (also see Streeck 1980). For example, the utterances "I command" display *and* accomplish the act of commanding.

3. Sacks, Schegloff, and Jefferson's (1974) turn-taking analysis assumes talk occurring in natural everyday interactions between equals in contexts where turn taking is spontaneous and turn allocation is free to vary. These researchers describe

a two-part structure in which a question receives an answer or a greeting receives a return greeting, and when it is not interrupted by side or insertion sequences, this response takes place in the next immediate turn at talk, providing a sequential organization of conversation. Labov and Fanshel (1977) have provided a structural outline of the psychotherapeutic interview as an interactional event involving the exchange of information in a routine manner with defined boundaries and expected behaviors.

4. His remark implies that having large breasts made the woman "all girl" as small breasts could not. If this patient had been a man, would such an anatomy-based remark have been applied to his manhood by a doctor checking his genitals for potentially cancerous lumps? The growing literature on doctors' differential treatment of female and male patients suggests that it would not (see Schiefelbein 1980).

5. Interestingly, David Silverman (1984), comparing National Health Service (NHS) care with private practice in England found the opposite. Once again health care delivery in the two settings was more similar than different, but private practice patients, as paying customers, exerted more control over the interaction. This difference may occur because, though most Americans are paying customers (albeit through a variety of insurance and aid), the imagery of the expert-layperson relationship has prevailed. In England, the emphasis on NHS makes the private patient the exception and thus more obvious as a paying customer.

6. Scheff discusses a similar situation when the psychiatrist asks the questions; the client answers. The psychiatrist's control of the interview puts him in the position to accept, reject, and ignore the client's answers while concomitantly "leading her to define the situation as one in which she is at fault" (1968:14).

7. By separating the social and contextual from the biomedical and technical as I do throughout the book, I do not intend to deny the social construction aspects of all of these categories. For it is a social-historical decision to assign technical or biomedical areas as such, dichotomized from the contextual, in the first place—a decision firmly embedded in modern Western culture. I separate them conceptually here for the sake of argument first to show how they are dichotomized in modern Western society and medicine and second (in later chapters) to examine such dichotomies as problematic.

8. Similarly, Fisher (1986) discusses how gynecological residents promote hysterectomies to women patients. She asserts that the doctors' selling techniques reflect self-interest rather than concern for women. Scully (1980) outlines the ways in which gynecological obstetric residents learn to persuade women to accept treatment procedures.

4 | Delusions in Discourse

The doctor can declare, "The patient doesn't have anything to say about it" within the confines of his or her office, but once outside this context, the situation is different. To begin to answer the questions raised at the end of the last chapter, I conducted in-depth interviews with women in their homes. I found that when asked and listened to, women had much to say. From their accounts a broader vision of reproduction as a social as well as a biological process emerges—a process inextricably entwined in women's daily lives and decision making. Although I asked questions and listened to responses, in these interviews women did most of the talking, discussing their sex lives, relationships, families, and work. When women's voices are listened to, one hears a story that echoes with the complex roles reproduction and sexuality play in their lives.[1]

Each woman, of course, reflected these concerns differently. Women's experiences are different because of many factors, including their class and race. The "generic" woman's experience is usually interpreted as that of a middle-class white woman. Inquiry into difference is rare. Although my study is too small to draw systematic conclusions about difference, I did observe two relevant trends. First, the darker a woman's skin and/or the lower her place on the economic scale, the poorer the care and efforts at explanation she received. Women of color and/or an economically poor background were more apt to be seen as "difficult" patients when they asked questions, were more likely to be urged to use birth control pills or the IUD rather than the diaphragm in the clinic, and in the private practitioner's office, where nearly all women received the pill, they were more likely to be talked down to, scolded, and patronized.

Second, despite these important differences, there were also similarities. Women's treatment was along a continuum whereby all women
received care that both reflected and reinforced society's definitions of and
attitudes toward women, their bodies, and reproduction. In the interviews, as well as in my informal talks with women, a general underlying
question, often only vaguely articulated, persisted. Although each woman's
question took a different form and encompassed unique circumstances,
there was discernible similarity or pattern in the concerns expressed. In
broad outline this question was "How can I more fully integrate my sexual
activity and reproductive needs with what I want from life? How can
these activities be more under my control?" Discussion about such questions was not encouraged in doctor-patient conversations, yet my interviews show them to be repeated concerns connected to contraception and
health. When women did try to raise variations on this theme with their
doctors, they were interrupted or cut off. Women accepted this truncation
of their social lives, accepting doctors' views that such topics were beyond
the scope of medical care. This dominance prevails not only in the doctor's
office but often in the women's understandings of their bodies once outside
the office. Rampant public discussion may address medical mistakes, ar-
rogance, and insensitivity, but the subtler side of the medical model goes
uncontested, indeed unnoticed by many.

METHOD

As a means of looking at these differing dynamics between what is discussed
in the doctor-patient interaction and what women willingly talked about
when encouraged to do so, a modified version of a sociolinguistic technique
called "text expansion" is useful. William Labov and David Fanshel (1977)
combine a linguist's respect for formal rules of discourse with a commitment to the social side of human interaction. Using snippets of a therapist-
client conversation (the opening fifteen minutes of the twenty-fifth therapy
session), they have developed a method of expanding the text and thereby
expanding our understanding of the structure and content of discourse.
Each segment of the discourse between therapist and client is expanded
upon with other sources of information to tell us more about the therapy
encounter, the model of treatment used, the client, and the therapist.

Although their approach has been applauded as an innovative addition to sociolinguistic analysis, they have also had their critics. Neither
Labov nor Fanshel was present during the therapy session, so they take
their expansions from notes in the client's chart and from discussions with
the therapist. They used playback sessions with the therapist to illuminate

the therapeutic process "from the subjective viewpoint of the therapist, enriched by her own theoretical orientation" (p. 5). There were no such sessions with the client. The researchers, in fact, were explicit in their desire to place themselves inside the psychiatric theoretical model. Their incorporation of social understandings into discourse analysis stops at the level of psychotherapy. Both the interpretations of clients and larger societal influences are left unexplored. Judy Sherer examines how, in ignoring these broader social issues, Labov and Fanshel bring an unexamined patriarchal bias to bear on their expansions of the talk:

> Notably *absent* from this collection of explicit sources is any theory about the material and ideational organization of the society in which they and the conversational participants are embedded. This absence does not mean, however, that no higher-level assumptions enter into their analysis. Labov and Fanshel necessarily rely on the knowledge they have acquired by virtue of their membership in a capitalist patriarchal culture. This knowledge, however, is not reflected upon; therefore, it enters the analysis only in the most implicit and indirect ways. (1979:22)

Sherer points out that by falling into the unexamined life, Labov and Fanshel's research conclusions suffer. The client's problems as well as our understanding of them are analyzed in the same mystified manner by therapist and researcher. The psychiatric medical model approach to social problems goes unquestioned.

The methodology employed by Labov and Fanshel's study is intricate and intriguing, despite criticisms. For my purposes here—better understanding of the doctor–female patient relationship—modification of this method is useful. First, I do not go into the depth Labov and Fanshel's detailed discourse analysis entails. My interest is in using a form of their methodology best suited to excavating the content rather than the form of the conversations. Second, my approach to the text is different. I have, so to speak, turned Labov and Fanshel on their heads. Since one of my interests is to bring historical, cultural, and institutional analyses to bear on understanding everyday interactions and events, discussion of these larger issues is an ever-present factor in the data analysis. Indeed, the data here are understandable only when viewed through a larger lens.

My emphasis within the data expansion is also different. Verbatim segments of the doctor-patient discourse are used in conjunction with verbatim segments of my in-depth interviews with patients. Rather than rely on doctors to explain women's behaviors, I have drawn on women's experiences to understand better their medical relationships. Expansion, the broadening of one piece of conversation with additional information, is provided here by the women's perspectives on their health and reproduction. Despite a shift in context of discourses (or perhaps because of it) from medical office to home environment, understandings of the *consequences* of medical events are broadened.

Throughout her writings on feminist methodologies, Dorothy Smith calls for close attention to the experiences of the people we study. Conceptual frameworks and analyses must take into account women's voices as a basis for feminist research. She points out, "Our conceptual procedures should be capable of explicating and analyzing the properties of their experienced world. . . . Their reality, their varieties of experience must be an unconditional datum" (1974:12). This datum provides yet another text for investigation.

The medical perspective has been well researched and all too often provided the sole datum. The model of medicine has been dissected, the medical educational process has been explored and deplored, doctors have been interviewed and have written detailed autobiographical accounts of their experiences from medical school through internship, residency, and so forth. There has been far less coverage of what patients' experiences tell us about the health care system. The data we do have records complex attitudes, predominantly negative, toward health care. In this chapter a more elusive issue is discussed. When doctor-patient interactions are expanded by excerpts from my interviews, a disjunctive picture emerges—one that both participants were unaware existed. The contrast becomes clear between the doctors' biomedical assumptions based on their physiological orientation to the body and women's contextual understandings based on knowledge of their social lives. It is the doctor's definitions that prevail. Of even more importance here is that medical dominance over the parameters of the interaction produces inadequate communication, which in turn leads to inadequate medical care—a lack that is seldom properly understood.

Elliot Mishler (1984) delineates two voices in the medical interview—the "voice of medicine" (biomedical, clinical information) and the "voice of the lifeworld" (social, contextual information). Although doctors and patients talk in both voices, doctors emphasize the former and patients are often concerned with the latter. Since doctors exert more control in the medical encounter, the "voice of medicine" represents the routine. The less often heard "voice of the lifeworld" represents but a breach in the normative flow of medical conversations.

Given the misunderstandings between participants to be discussed in the following data, the medical model, based on its own knowledge system, is in danger of short-circuiting itself. Good technical care, the domain of modern medicine, is put at risk at its most crucial intersection—communication between doctors and patients. It is at this intersection that

	Patient	Doctor
PATTERN 1	Has relevant information and tries to express it	Interrupts patient
PATTERN 2	Unaware; does not try to express information	Has relevant information; withholds information
PATTERN 3	Has relevant information; withholds information	Unaware; does not try to express information

FIGURE 1.
Categorization for information exchange between doctor and patient

women's voices and medical care all too often pass each other by. Organizational differences in the two settings influenced communication, but the problems to be discussed here were similar in the clinic and private practice office: *often what the patient really needed to talk about was ignored in medical encounters.* This gap between patients' and doctors' perspectives took three main forms.

In the first pattern, the discourse displayed women trying to direct topics in the medical encounter. Women inserted their views or tried to raise their concerns about aspects of their lives important to contraceptive use and decision making but were cut off by their doctors. In the second pattern, women did not press their views or concerns. It appears as if they were unaware that their information might contribute to or change the understanding of their problems, and doctors did little to change this view. In the third pattern, women had their own agenda, which did not emerge in discussions with the doctors. Patients withheld information about their contraceptive needs from unaware doctors.

Whatever the pattern of the medical interaction, expansion of the interviews highlighted topics that were relevant to, but absent from, the discussion of contraceptive choice. These topics included technical information but centered around contextual, social parts of women's lives and were generally defined by doctors and accepted by women as inappropriate in medical discourse. In informal conversations all of the doctors in this study expressed boredom, irritation, or both with women who tried to "tell me her life story."[2]

I will discuss the patterns separately, highlighting each with two examples. I examined all of the transcripts in detail to draw out recurrent themes and patterns. Once I identified these patterns, I chose a small sample to illustrate themes that appear in the data. Thus the six examples discussed in this chapter exemplify findings from the twenty taped interviews I conducted with the same women I taped talking with their doctors. It is important, however, to remember that the patterns can either overlap or show up in the same interview and are, at best, rough measures for varying and complex dynamics.

THE DOCTOR-PATIENT DISCOURSE AND EXPANSION OF THE TEXT

PATTERN 1:

Women attempt to express their concerns in the medical interaction—doctors cut off their attempts

Maria Martinez

Let us return to materials introduced in the beginning of Chapter 3. Maria Martinez is twenty-six, married, and has a tired air about her which can easily turn to animated interest if her lively sense of humor is aroused. She has four children ranging in age from eleven years to six months and a varied contraceptive history. The clinic rarely recommends the IUD for birth control, but it has been recommended to Maria because she has four children and the clinic feels this is enough for a low-income (Medicaid) family. She also has had a history of unexpected pregnancy, which places her in the clinic's category of an inept contraceptor. Maria has, somewhat reluctantly, agreed to this birth control method. Her past experience with the IUD has not been satisfactory. On this visit she comes to the doctor for the standard pre-IUD check-up, and an appointment is made for insertion of the IUD in two weeks.

Doctor (D)-Patient (P) Discourse

> P: It won't hurt will it?
> D: Oh, I doubt it.
> P: I'm taking your word (laugh).
> D: I haven't had anybody pass out from one yet.
> P: The last time/
> D: (cuts patient off with a joke; both patient and doctor laugh)
> P: The last time when I had that Lippes Loop, oh, God/
> D: (interrupts patient)/You won't even know what's going on. We'll just
slip that in and you'll be so busy talking and you won't know it.

In the doctor-patient discourse Maria asks a direct question about possible pain. In two subsequent turns she tries to raise her past and painful experience with the IUD. Each time she is interrupted and cut off by the doctor. She attempts to raise the topic three times. This makes her an assertive patient. Most women in this study did not raise topics but merely responded to them.

Medical literature supports the view that women experience pain with insertion of the IUD rather than after it is in place. The doctor seems to assume this to be the case with Maria as well. This was not Maria's concern. My follow-up interview provides an expansion of what Maria was trying to express.

Expansion of the Text

P: I tried an IUD. . . . I got an IUD put in, a Lippes Loop (interviewer [I]: Uh huh), and I got that put in and I had that in August, for four months and I couldn't take it.

I: Well, what was it like using the IUD?

P: Oh, God, it was the most awful, terriblest, uncomfortable, it was awful. I hated it. . . . I had it taken out 'cause I couldn't hack it. . . .

I: How come?

P: I, it, it killed me. I was, oh, oh, that's why I'm so scared with this one, the one I'm going to get. . . . I remember the pain, yeah, it was awful.

I: When it was put in?

P: No, when it was put in it didn't hurt. . . . It was okay all month long until I started my period, like the day before I started my period, my God in heaven, I'd be on the bed crying in pain. . . . I even started taking pain killers.

I: Why did you keep it?

P: Because when I went, I went to the Public Health . . . and they just said . . . you'll have a little cramp and that's it. And you know that actually it didn't hurt a bit getting it in. (I: Uh huh.) It didn't bother me a bit, but it was just that I was so scared and tense (I: Uh huh), and nobody would tell you, relax, and, you know, take it easy, or anything like that. Let you just freak out, you know, you just, then it was fine, you know, nothing bothered me. Went back to school that day and everything. And then the next month when my period started, well, the doctor had told me, "now don't be a baby and come back because you get a little pain." (I: Uh huh.) "Don't be a big baby and come back and say you want it out. You gotta give it a couple of months chance." So I kept saying, oh, it's just getting adjusted, it's just getting, the first time, it's just, you know, just the pain, it's just going to get adjusted. (I: Oh.) The next month, it was "don't be a baby Maria," they said "don't be a baby; hmm, hmm, hmm."

The doctor made an assumption regarding Maria's concerns based on a generalized understanding of IUD use. Maria's experiences, however, are particularistic, based on her own history of pain after insertion. Conflict in perspective and the doctor's more powerful position to control the discourse left her concerns unaddressed. In turn, the fears the doctor assumed she was addressing (pain on insertion) were lightheartedly dismissed.

Corinne Conrad

Corinne Conrad is a divorced woman in her late twenties. She has short blond hair and is shy and tentative in her speech as if she is never quite sure she is saying the right thing. She is presently working as a dental assistant to support herself and her four-year-old daughter, Jenny. Corinne came to the clinic in December for two reproductive-related concerns— although now sexually inactive, she wanted birth control in case she might need it, and she has not had a menstrual period since the previous January (amenorrhea).

Doctor-Patient Discourse

> *D:* Okay, and your last period was when?
> *P:* Uhm, in January. . . .
> *D:* You haven't had a period since then?
> *P:* No, I, I went to a doctor, I think it was in July, and he gave me a shot to get it started and I had some spotting but it only lasted for a half a day and that was it. . . .
> *D:* Uhm, we could give you birth control pills to try to regulate your period.
> *P:* Well, I tried that, too, the doctor suggested it and I took them and they didn't, it didn't start either. . . .
> *D:* Uhm (pause).
> *P:* In January my husband and I were having difficulties and then we separated at the end of February/
> *D:* (interrupts)/Okay. But it's been almost a year/
> *P:* /Yeah, I know/
> *D:* /now since you had a period.

The doctor leaves the room to consult with another doctor.

> *D:* It would probably be a good idea to give you a test dose of this progesterone to see if you have a withdrawal bleeding. I assume that this is probably what you were injected with earlier this summer. . . . It would be uhm, the best idea to give you the progesterone for five days, have a withdrawal bleed, and then start you on the pill.

Corinne has not menstruated for one year—from the time she and her husband "were having difficulties." She raises this problem with the doctor, who brushes over the topic with a statement that implies a year is long enough to recover from a divorce. Although there may or may not be a causal link between Corinne's marital upset and her amenorrhea, her tentative raising of the issue expresses this as a concern. The doctor ignores this information and offers technical solutions in the form of progesterone and birth control pills, both of which have been tried in the past and failed.

Expansion of the Text

> *P:* Most of the time even before I had Jenny, I stayed at home because we did move a lot and we, or he would take leave and so we could just pack up and travel (I: Uh huh), so I never worked. . . . And then when he came back from overseas, we came out here and for the first six months that we were out here, we were very happy and content, and then after that, I just wanted to have

another child, but he kept saying no, but never gave me any reasons (I: Uh huh). And then after a long time it finally came to him, and he said he didn't love me any more and wanted a divorce.

I: Uh huh, and so how was, how did you feel about that?

P: I was rather upset. I, you know, I never expected it. He was going through a change, I noticed last fall and winter, but he was in the service for ten years and got out this April, and I thought it was just, uh, all the decision of getting out, going on to school, going on to medicine, you know, and there were financial concerns, and I thought that's his major cau . . . or worry (I: Uh huh), at that time (I: Uh huh), but then he finally came to me and said he didn't know how he felt about me any more. He thought he didn't love me. . . .

I: And did he have any reasons for, for this change toward you. . . ?

P: Well, he really wouldn't talk about it. . . . He just said he was going through a change. . . . The way I was brought up in the, in the community or my father and mother's (I: Uh huh), relationship, because I was brought up in the Midwest and it seems like people back there are more family oriented and I was like programmed, you know, when you grow up, you're going to get married and have your family. . . . Uhm, I'm very happy to be in the home situation, the family around me, and I enjoy doing things for someone special. . . .

I: Yes, uh huh. So you, you mentioned something about stopping your periods. You want to talk a little bit about that?

P: Okay, in January of this year my, I was on the pill at the time, and my period stopped.

I: Even while you were on the pill?

P: Right. And then in February I still didn't get one and we separated and so finally in March, I went in and had a pregnancy test run just to make sure [it was negative].

Once again we see a woman volunteering information about her life that she feels is pertinent to her health. She is a woman who holds traditional values, she has been divorced unexpectedly without understanding why, and a year later she is no happier with this decision than she was when it took place. Corinne makes a tentative connection between her reproductive processes and her social circumstances. Her doctor, well trained in the biomedical model, focuses on biological processes severed from the social events of her life. Both of the above women represent a pattern in medical encounters in which the patient has a story to tell but is not allowed to tell it.

PATTERN 2:
Women are unaware that they need more information—doctors withhold information

Marylou Long

Marylou Long is a single woman in her mid-thirties. She runs the "one-girl" office for her father's construction firm and takes classes in Spanish and real estate at the local community night college. She was originally put on the birth control pill in her teens to regulate her periods, and in her late twenties when she became sexually active she resumed taking the pill as a contraceptive method. She went to her private practitioner in September for a checkup because her menstrual periods stopped in June and for a renewal prescription for the pill.

Doctor-Patient Discourse

D: So you haven't menstruated since June.
P: Yeah, I don't think I did in July. I'm pretty sure I didn't. . . .
D: Okay, you haven't missed any pills?
P: No.
D: Look, what I think is happening, that your pills are not strong enough, you know? I've put you on a very low pill as you know . . . and sometimes this will cause (swallows word). Now what I would like to do is when you finish your pills, let's see, you're on the twenty-eight days. (long pause)
P: Right. Uh, twenty-one day.
D: Twenty-one day, all right. When you finish your pills, and if you don't menstruate within five to six days, come in. I'll give you an injection to get you started.
P: Okay.
D: If you do menstruate, come in then. . . . I will give you a prescription for a different kind. . . .
P: Right, uh hum.

The doctor suggests as a solution to Marylou's amenorrhea an injection (progesterone) and a stronger birth control pill. She seems to accept this treatment plan unquestioningly. The doctor and Marylou seem to agree. Despite this agreement there is argument in the medical community as to the safety and efficacy of this treatment for amenorrhea,[3] as well as a disinclination for the stronger hormonal content pills—information that does not emerge in this encounter.

Expansion of the Text

I: Uhm, do you talk to, have you ever talked to someone about birth control?
P: Not besides the doctor, no.

Later in the interview we discussed the amount of information received from doctors on contraception:

P: Not a lot. Uhm, a little bit with Dr. M but not, you know, not a, specific.
I: And how did you decide on using the pill as a method?
P: Uh, it's the most convenient and it's most reliable.
I: Do you ever worry at all about the health side effects or any of/
P: /Well, it's a concern but I uhm, I've never had any side effects at all

from it (I: Uh huh). And I go in, I go in to the doctor twice a year and I know he knows what he's doing, so, you know, I feel reasonably safe, you know . . . safe with it. I'm sure there's a chance but there is with anything. . . .

    I: Okay, and how about any long-term, have you had any long-term experiences, relationships with men?

    P: Ah, let's see, not really long term.

    I: How about the man you were talking about that you broke up with in December?

    P: Well, we were together for about six weeks but that was the time he was here. . . . I haven't had a boyfriend, you know, an actual boyfriend, I mean I've had occasionally, you know, had something, someone that just didn't work out but I haven't had a boyfriend since then.

    I: Uhm, so have you ever had sexual relations on a regular basis?

    P: Well, when I've got a boyfriend, yes.

The expansion provides a picture of a woman who for nine months has had very sporadic sexual activity, no regular "boyfriend," and no anticipation of regular sexual activity on the horizon. Given the medical controversy over appropriate treatment for amenorrhea, the medical questioning of the high estrogen dosage in the stronger birth control pills, and Marylou's present reduced sexual activity, a fuller discussion of the range of contraceptive options was called for. Alternative methods were never discussed, and Marylou's stated reasons for using the pill mirror nearly exactly Dr. M's choice of words when recommending this method to new patients. This is not to say that Marylou should *never* use oral contraception, but her decision should be an informed one. An alternative contraceptive method might have helped her health, but neither the doctor nor Marylou brought it up as a possibility. Is this the equal responsibility of the two participants? I think not. Doctors have historically fought to be the dispensers of knowledge on health in general and contraception in particular. Given the asymmetry in the relationship at this time, the greater responsibility in our model of health care falls on the doctor. This responsibility is reflected in Marylou's reliance (perhaps overreliance) on her doctor as her sole source of contraceptive information.

Maria Martinez

Let us return to the medical interaction with Maria Martinez (Pattern 1) to see how the various patterns can appear in different parts of the same interview. The doctors in the clinic generally present to women a very long, negative oration on the IUD and a low-key push for the birth control pill (for example, Chapter 3, Example 14). In this case, however, the IUD has already been recommended. The doctor raises one question in the interview which indicates his general preference for the pill over the IUD. Maria's answer terminates any further inquiry in this direction. Maria's response does provide active direction to the medical interaction. She is not, however, consciously trying to raise issues as she was earlier with her questions on IUD insertion (Pattern 1).

Doctor-Patient Discourse

D: Uh hum. What's the pill do for you?
P: Oh, they're okay except I uh, you gotta remember how to take them.
D: True, true (initiates pre-IUD exam).

Both Maria and the doctor assume that she cannot use the birth control pill because she implies that in the past she has forgotten to take it. In fact, it is her lack of remembrance that has convinced the clinic staff that Maria needs an IUD. The doctor, having no information on Maria's social history except that she had trouble remembering to take the pill at one time and had an unexpected pregnancy as a result, proceeds with what he considers to be the most dangerous form of birth control—the IUD. He thinks it dangerous, Maria is afraid of it, yet it has been selected as the method of choice.

From this medical interaction one is likely to deduce that there are only two contraceptive methods available—the IUD and the pill. This is obviously not the case; however, there is no mention of alternatives. The clinic predominantly prescribed the pill, dispensed many diaphragms, and rarely suggested IUDs, condoms, and/or foam. Birth control pills or IUDs, however, were the main methods considered appropriate for a woman labeled a "birth control failure."

Expansion of the Text

I: How long did you use the pill?
P: Uh, let me see (inaudible) uh, two years. . . .
I: What was it like using this method?
P: Back then it was okay, because I could remember to take them. . . .
I: How come you got off of it [birth control pills]?
P: I can't remember. I guess I just, me and my husband were fighting a lot and we started fighting a lot and then we separated and I just didn't take it. I said, well I don't need them.
I: And then what happened?
P: I did need it.
I: Then what happened?
P: Michael [patient's son].
I: All right, and so, did you get on birth control after he was born?
P: Yeah . . . the pill again [husband returned].
I: Okay, and for how long did you use that pill?
P: Four years, almost five years. . . . At first it was, about the first two years it was okay, but then I, I don't know what went wrong in my head or anything, but I, I kept forgetting to take them. . . . I'd forget to take them and then I'd, I'd, you know, get scared every month. . . . And I didn't even get preg-

nant, you know, and then when I, about the last year, I realized I really wanted a baby, you know, and I didn't take them, [birth control pills] and I didn't get pregnant. You know, I wouldn't get, I tried so hard . . . you know, my husband kept saying 'oh no, no no.' . . . I wanted to get pregnant and I knew that if I just got pregnant, that he wouldn't say nothing. You know he'd be happy and everything (I: Uh huh). But I wouldn't get pregnant. . . . What the hell's wrong with me? I'd do it every day for a month. . . . I kept it scheduled in my purse calendar. "I did it today—X—I did it today . . . one whole month and I didn't get pregnant. And I thought, why, how is this possible. . . . I just felt that I may never be able to have another baby. . . . And in January, I got pregnant [nearly one year later, by which time Ms. M had decided against another baby].

    I: What kind of birth control were you using?

    P: Nothing.

    I: How come?

    P: Because I hadn't been using it. I thought I wa—, I couldn't get pregnant, I hadn't been using it in so long . . . I didn't think I was ever going to get pregnant again.

Maria's social history with the birth control pill is confusing to her and unknown to the doctor. She has used oral contraceptives both successfully and unsuccessfully. While forgetting to take the pill, she came to realize she wanted another child and actively stopped taking the pill. She does not understand why she did not get pregnant. She did not realize that it can take up to a year after using oral contraceptives to become fertile. Thus Maria tried to become pregnant and did not. She decided she was sterile, did not use birth control, became pregnant, and was labeled a birth control failure in need of an IUD by the clinic. From Maria's birth control pill history, it seems possible that she took the pill regularly when she did not want to become pregnant and "forgot" (unconsciously and consciously) to take it with some regularity when she did want another child (see Luker 1975 for reproductive decision making and contraceptive use).

    Once again none of this history is explored in the medical interaction. The definition of Maria as an incompetent user of birth control is based on a slim and misleading view lacking contextual information about her contraceptive history. The doctor, whose responsibility it is to gather information relative to the decision-making process, does not explore contextual issues. Contraception as medically defined is a technical topic, not a contextual one. When social information is used by the doctor, as in this case, he draws on an abstract, stereotypic view that when women are poor and have a history of unplanned pregnancy, they are inept contraceptors.

    Viewed from another perspective, doctors are inept. I never heard doctors explain to women, when prescribing the pill, the possibility of temporary infertility if they stopped using this method. This was explained if women came to the doctors to stop the pill, but many women, like Maria, stop on their own. When such basic information is not forthcoming from doctors, the results can be devastating. Thus Maria did not have the benefit of a helpful discussion with the doctor on the contextual aspects of her birth control choice (not expected in the medical model), nor had she, in the past, been given the technical information she needed to understand her own reproductive processes (information to be expected in the medical model).

Maria herself had not examined her own reproductive history enough to introduce contextual issues that were relevant to her contraceptive choice. Indeed, she accepted the parameters of the medical interview within both the doctor-patient interaction and her own consciousness about birth control. This case is a further example of how such a narrow treatment model can be misleading for all the participants, but it is women who pay the price. Maria, labeled a poor contraceptive user, was denied a full discussion of all the birth control options.[4] A fuller explanation of the possibilities and a clearer understanding of her own history would at least have left her in a position to choose a method, rather than settle for the clinic's choice. In other parts of our interview it became clear that Maria was confused about the barrier methods. She thought a diaphragm had to be inserted just before intercourse, like a condom. In fact, Maria was particularly susceptible to the clinic's persuasion because she had accepted its verdict of her contraceptive irresponsibility.

In sum, both Marylou Long and Maria Martinez are representative of women who are unaware that they need a range of information that is not forthcoming. Doctors, having been taught that they know best, make decisions based on stereotypic attitudes toward women's behavior (as in the case of Maria's unplanned pregnancy) and a technical fix for contraception (as in the case of Marylou).

PATTERN 3:
Women withhold information—doctors are unaware

Amanda Adams

Amanda Adams is a college senior at a large university and majors in environmental design. She is twenty-one years old and is affiliated with a popular sorority on campus. Her appearance, exuding youthful exuberance, brings to mind "now generation" television advertisements. She came to her private practitioner for a routine checkup and a birth control pill prescription renewal.

Doctor-Patient Discourse

D: Pills are doing all right?
P: Yup. . . .
D: Uh, Amanda, I'm going to give you a six months supply. . . . Uh, look,

uh, if I shouldn't be here or something then you're stuck, always when you start the last package, uh get in touch. . . . You're taking these twenty-one days, you prefer those to the twenty-eight?

P: Yeah.

D: How do you buy your pills? Do you buy just one at a time?

P: Two months, two months at a time.

D: When you get the last two [birth control pill packages], you know, then on the last one, take a red pencil and mark across it, across, and then you know this is my last package, you know. . . . Here are your happy pills. Don't miss them. Anything unforeseen, you let me know, you know. You know, you read the pamphlet, you know the potential risks are minimal but you are aware of them.

P: Uh hum.

Amanda comes to the doctor's office, goes through a gynecological examination, tells the doctor the pills are doing fine, and leaves with a renewal prescription. This doctor believes the birth control pill is the best contraceptive method for the majority of women and assumes that Amanda concurs. On this premise, the doctor prescribes "happy pills" for the patient, leaving little opening for a discussion to emerge on alternative methods.

Expansion of the Text

P: I want to get off of it [the pill] for the time being, let my body system take over for a while and let it get back on its own because I'm scared something could happen. . . .

I: /What kinds of things?

P: Oh just, having problems when you do want to get pregnant (I: Uh huh), because your body won't ovulate when you, you know, when it's supposed, you know what I mean, it's it's triggered. . . .

I: So you're going to, you're thinking of getting off of it for a while?

P: Yeah. . . . I plan to get off of it because I'm kinda ify-ify but I do think there's side effects to it when you stay on it too long. . . . Especially now since Bill and I aren't really going out that much anyways.

I: Yeah, and what kind of birth control method do you think you would use then?

P: I have no idea, I have no idea. I have no background and I'd have to find out.

I: And have you talked to Dr. M about that?

P: No. . . . I just feel strange talking to him. It's just the way I was brought up, you know, a male. . . . I, I've honestly wished, I could find a lady gynecologist and when I do I hate to say it, but I will transfer, not because he's not a good doctor because he's an excellent doctor (I: Uh huh). . . . [But] you just don't let a male see you like that, you, until you're fully dressed, and so this, after that being pounded into my head for twenty-one years, this, it's just not. . . . I mean he just makes me feel uncomfortable. . . .

I: Uh hum, and you feel that that's true, would be true of any male doctor, or/

P: /Yeah, obviously, yeah.

Amanda finds herself in the paradox of needing information she is too uncomfortable to elicit from the one place authorized to dispense it. The expansion reveals, first, that she is nervous about her health and future fertility on the pill, second, that the relationship with her boyfriend, Bill, has slowed down and she finds she does not need constant birth control, and third, that she has no idea about what method she would use in place of the pill. Because the doctor is a man, she is uncomfortable asking him for information. Her efforts to find a woman doctor yielded little help. The number of female gynecologists is still relatively small; the ones she did call had long waiting lists or were taking no new patients. Furthermore, once women gynecologists are found, there is no guarantee that they will offer a different model of health care. When I suggested the university clinic, which would be free and available, Amanda was appalled. To go to a school-affiliated office would risk others knowing about her sexual activity, which she did not reveal to her friends or sorority.

Amanda exemplifies a dilemma many women face in the gynecologist's office. Society says good women keep their bodies to themselves until marriage (or sexual intimacy). Sexual organs are not to be revealed to strangers of the opposite sex. Yet doctors are often strangers or, at best, office acquaintances. Emerson (1970) discusses strategies doctors and their staff use to manage this breach in social rules. Even with careful management, however, this discomfort can add yet another dimension to the distance and communication gap between doctor and patient.

Sally Barrett

Sally Barrett is a woman in her mid-twenties, assistant manager of a bank, married with no children and no immediate plans to have any. She came to the private practitioner for a postabortion checkup and for birth control. The doctor gave her a birth control pill prescription at the time of her abortion, and today he renews her prescription for the next three months.

Doctor-Patient Discourse

D: You take your pills?
P: Uh hum, I still have some, maybe a week's worth.
D: I'm going to give you today a prescription for three months.
P: Okay.
D: Then I want you here when you start on the last package.
P: Okay. . . .
D: Okay? Do you read the pamphlet uh in the, well, which comes with the pills, huh?
P: Okay (nodding head).
D: And, you know, there are certain risks but you're at risk when you cross the street too. . . . All right, you dress, come and see me. I will give you a prescription, you know, and everything is fine.

But everything is not fine. As in the previous case, the doctor prescribes a method of contraception to a woman, who, it turns out, is reluctant.

Expansion of the Text

I: What was it like using the pill during that, that time?

P: It was all right. I didn't, the only physical side effect I had at that point was uh the splotchy skin, the colasma. . . . Uhm, I hated those and I got them pretty bad. . . .

I: Where were the, where were the blotchy, the blotchy skin?

P: On my face. . . . It was my own personal vanity. They were pretty dark and they were pretty definite, and it looked like I had a moustache and (I: Uh huh), uh, it looked, I had them around on my cheeks and they were pretty definite. My, I didn't, make-up wouldn't cover them up or anything like that, and I never had very good skin to begin with and I didn't need to add something like that to it. . . .

I: Okay, and uhm why did you switch to the diaphragm?

P: I think it was, my sister-in-law was using a diaphragm at the time. . . . I thought I'd give it a try (I: Uh huh, okay), and I'm still using it. . . .

I: And when you were at Dr. M's office . . . he talked to you about being on the pill . . . and you didn't mention the diaphragm?

P: Yeah. He's pretty strong hearted and uh about that, and uh/

I: /About what?

P: Taking the pill. . . . He's been after me to take it for a while and every time that I say no, he just looks at me. . . . He's uh, he's set in his ways and so uh, the, we've had the same discussion over and over.

I: And have you tried telling him, talking to him about the fact that you, you just aren't going to use it?

P: Yeah, uhm, and he'll ask my concerns (I: Uh huh), and he assures me that my age, uh is a safety factor there. Uhm, I don't know . . . that it's good. There's a lot of things that have come up about oh, clotting of blood and different things and there's a lot being tested that's so unknown, you know. . . . I think he's a good doctor, but instead of working with me, uh with the diaphragm, he'd rather see me take the pill . . . and so instead of getting into confrontations with him, because he's pretty strong willed . . . but uh he's doing it for my own good.

Like Maria Martinez, Sally Barrett has been labeled a "birth control failure" (she has had an abortion), which could account for the doctor's adamance about the pill. When this doctor (like the majority of gynecologists) prescribes and recommends the pill as the most effective nonsurgical form of birth control for women, the tendency is to minimize the dangers with such statements as "you're at risk when you cross the street too"—a statement often mirrored in patients' discourse (see Marylou Long). But Sally is concerned about the safety of the birth control pill and has suffered ill effects using this method in the past.

Interestingly, although Sally would prefer to have the doctor work with her on using the diaphragm, she still feels he is basically a good doctor who looks out for her best interests. This is a good example of the basic conflict between trying to retain a trust for the doctor while concomitantly refusing his advice.

If one were to witness this doctor-patient interaction or listen to a tape of it, one would surmise that Sally was using an oral contraceptive. Her view of this method does not emerge in the encounter. Rather, she purposely withholds information from the doctor, whom she has come to and is paying for a service, to avoid an old and repeated confrontation about her reproductive control. Although this is evidence of active participation on Sally's part, it signifies an unequal relationship. The power to choose is covertly managed by the patient. The doctor's overt control in the interaction goes uncontested.

Both Amanda Adams and Sally Barrett are examples of women who are uncomfortable enough with their medical care to conceal information from their doctors. Doctors, understandably unaware of withheld concerns, do not in general probe for the information concealed here.

REFLECTIONS ON THE DATA

The medical profession has two conflicting goals with respect to delivering contraceptive services. First, the health care system is committed to help women control the reproductive function. Second, the system is organized to promote health. Doctors are caught between these two interests. At the present time, the major forms of contraception are technically efficient in that they allow sexual activity freer from risk of unwanted pregnancy than at any time in history. At the same time, these methods can create havoc for women's health. In Chapter 1, David Hilfiker was quoted on his dilemma as a physician of continually being at risk of harming people. Doctors prescribing modern methods of birth control must assume that they will harm some women.[5] Perhaps the known benefits do outweigh the potential risks. On this conclusion the jury is still out, however, and the contradiction between the two aims of medicine remains.[6]

The medical profession is in the position of prescribing treatments to healthy women that can make them unhealthy, creating a paradox for women as well as doctors. Both doctors and patients are caught between the two interests—controlling reproduction and remaining healthy—with doctors generally responding predominantly to the former, often at cost to the latter. Women in my data were concerned with both. They needed to control their reproduction but did not want to do so at a cost to their health. Yet they often did not have much to say in the medical interactions. When they did contribute information, it was often in the form of stories or social commentaries deemed inappropriate to the issues at hand.

But women's stories, as we have seen, are important for reproductive control and adequate health care. In fact, it is in these stories that the two sides of the conflict between reproductive control and health could meet. More careful, informed choice on the part of patients could heighten contraceptive efficacy and decrease the health risks.

Maria Martinez's history with the IUD is extremely negative. The doctor's misunderstanding of her fears, and his interruption of her attempts to correct his impression, leave these fears unexplored. Furthermore, none of the less dangerous barrier methods were discussed. Maria's history of birth control use when examined contextually provides a different picture of her contraceptive competence and makes alternative methods plausible. She left the clinic after this exam and did not return because by the time for her next appointment she felt too afraid of the IUD. She and her husband had resumed using condoms—a method she found distasteful. She felt reproductively insecure and sexually turned off by condoms, feelings that contributed to a sexual withdrawal, resulting in her concern for her own sexuality and marital friction. These dynamics represent a pattern in which unaware doctors discourage medical discussions with patients, thus limiting women's abilities to evaluate their options and control their lives.

Corinne Conrad received a technical fix—a progesterone shot and birth control pills—that failed to make her menstruate this time as it had failed the first time. When I conducted a telephone interview (follow-up to the in-depth interview) with her, she was depressed and felt she had nowhere to turn. She had accepted the doctor's definition that the problem was a physiological one in need of a medical cure, but she saw no reason to return to the clinic. Her treatments, in her view, both with a previous doctor and with the doctor in the clinic, had been useless. Both Maria Martinez and Corinne Conrad chose at least temporarily to "drop out" of the medical system. Their dilemma, however, was where to turn for the help they needed. Even if they had the money or time to explore, they had no idea where to look.

Amanda Adams and Sally Barrett represent women who do not consider abandoning their doctor visits. They just are not able to use them in the most productive manner. Amanda Adams needed information she was too shy to ask for from a male physician. One hopes she found this information elsewhere. Whether it was given adequately and in time to affect her reproductive choices is an open question.

Sally Barrett tried to interact with her physician in an open way, found this uncomfortable, and decided to manipulate the encounter. She and her doctor disagree. Though she blames herself for being vain, the blotchy skin did bother her. She is also worried about more general effects of the pill. Her concerns are not unreasonable. Most of us would be concerned about large, distinct changes in skin color for cosmetic and health reasons. Further, the negative evidence on the pill is certainly worthy of consideration. Sally comes to the doctor for a service, pays him a considerable fee to help her regulate her reproduction (thus help her control her life), and finds she has to withhold information to have his cooperation. Such an interaction is the antithesis of what good reproductive health care should be.

Marylou Long, with her new, stronger birth control pills, represents women who are completely and complacently satisfied with their treatments. There is, however, question as to whether she should be. She is given a high-dosage estrogen pill as a treatment for a problem the medical profession is in conflict over and basically does not know much about. The controversial nature of this treatment is not discussed with her. Her contraceptive needs at this time are minimal, and if her present situation were made a part of the medical interaction, perhaps another approach could have been taken.

Although the gynecological specialty is supposed to deliver technical health care for bodily problems, the women in this study have not received even adequate technical care. This can be observed on two levels. First, by not presenting women with detailed discussion of all of their contraceptive options, physicians do not provide enough technical information for them to make informed decisions. Whether patients sought advice (as in Maria Martinez's attempts with the IUD), or remained unaware of this need (as in the case of Marylou Long), doctors were remiss. Second, doctors make contraceptive decisions on technical bases or abstract social assumptions (once a birth control failure, always a birth control failure), whereas women tend to think about these issues in personal, contextual terms. Given the doctors' more powerful position in the interactions, it is the medical interpretation that takes precedence. But as the analyses show, the exclusion of contextual information makes it harder for doctors and women to arrange even technical health care adequately.

The doctors and the patients are implicitly in conflict in these interactions. *Women come to doctors for help in understanding how to adjust their bodies to their social lives. Doctors' technical answers assume that women should adjust their social lives to their bodies.* The asymmetrical relationship between doctors and patients in our current medical model negates the possibility of open communication that would allow the doctors' technical expertise and the patients' contextual knowledge equal status, allowing participatory decision making. Doctors' concentration on bodily parts (the voice of medicine)—cells, ovaries, and uteri—offers generalizable and objective foci for gynecological study and practice. Contextual lives (the voice of the lifeworld) are seen as messy. Social information is complicated, subjective, and individual. Furthermore, to delve into such topics moves away from doctors' expertise and therefore necessitates more active participation on the part of the patients. In these areas patients have more knowledge than doctors. Such equality is often resisted by the medical profession. But just as doctors are technical experts, women (people) must become contextual experts in the medical encounter if the conflict between reproductive control and health is to be resolved.

The call to incorporate social, contextual information into contraceptive and health care decision making, however, presents a double-edged sword. I have argued that social, contextual information integrated with the physiological is crucial to adequate health care delivery, particularly for reproductive issues. In the data from my research, and studies mentioned earlier, people's perspectives and storytelling abilities are important for adequate care. Historically, however, the medical establishment has broadened its power base by assimilating aspects of the social into the medical. Given the hierarchical nature of our society and health care system, access to contextual, personal history allows those in authority to exert even more control. Patients' expertise could be co-opted. For example, Waitzkin's (1983) data on doctor-patient interactions reveal how when doctors do delve into the contextual, they use this information to exert more control, regulating behavior to maintain the status quo rather than meet people's needs. The Boston Women's Health Book Collective, in the *New Our Bodies, Ourselves* (1985), stresses the need for keeping doctors out of women's personal lives, where they all too often use social information to reinforce stereotypic sex roles. And as is shown in my own data, doctors' social talk (Chapter 3) does exactly that.

Thus it is not enough just to expand communication strategies. Rather, I am suggesting that along with adding contextual information to the current structure of the doctor-patient relationship, this relationship itself needs to be redefined in a more egalitarian way. Such a redefinition extends from the interactions themselves to larger socioeconomic and political contexts. Understanding medical relationships, like people's health concerns, requires contextual analyses.

CONCLUSION

In the current medical model, reproduction has been medicalized—the complexities are treated in a narrow disease model. When the social is raised by doctors it is done so in a detrimental way. For example, women's problems are "all in their heads," or women are seen first and foremost as reproducers. Furthermore, women's stories are either ignored or used against them. For example, Corinne Conrad, who suspects that her amenor-rhea may be connected to her divorce, faces being either interrupted, as in her interaction with this doctor, or being told yes, it is all psychosomatic, and thus dismissed without proper care. Health care is an either/or propo-sition in this system rather than a blending of the psychosocial with the biotechnical. Neither option helps people understand their bodies in light of their own experiences. Here lies the greatest dilemma. The subtlety of these dynamics, and the lack of awareness by doctors and patients of their existence, present the gravest risk. Not only are women's concerns trun-cated, but the medical definitions of reproduction mystify the issues, mak-ing it even more difficult for women to see clearly these issues and to create deeper understanding or alternate definitions. The power of the medical model is such that people (both doctors and patients) accept medical defi-nitions, both social and technical.

The medical encounter needs to involve two experts—doctor and pa-tient (necessitating a redefinition of the very word *patient*). This is both rare and difficult to achieve. The political-economic structure of American society and the institution of medicine are well entrenched and resistant to change. Doctors have grown accustomed to the role of expert. The profit motive and a commitment to a class-based, hierarchically arranged social order with strong power groups are tenaciously guarded. Sexist and racist assumptions are equally well entrenched and often unconsciously taken for granted in daily interactions. For people in need of health care, these larger factors directly affect the quantity and quality of the care they re-ceive. Carol Gilligan's (1982) analysis of women's psychological develop-ment shows how socialization into gender roles can further contribute to the ways in which women communicate with their doctors—behaviors that fit so well with the "good patient" role but do not necessarily contrib-ute to women's welfare.

Current research provides much evidence that sexism, elitism, and racism, as well as the patient role, all contribute to an inequality between doctors and women. Such analyses are especially helpful for understand-ing the data presented in Chapter 3 and certainly flavor the data presented in this chapter as well. But these views are not enough—too many ques-tions are left unanswered.

NOTES

1. Like medical interactions, interviews between social scientists and respon-dents are unequal, with topics directed by the interviewer. Aware of this inequality, I asked questions from the general to the specific. The women did the majority of

the talking, and I tried to keep interruptions to a minimum. I asked a new question only when the respondent stopped answering the first question. I went to the women's homes, was on a first name basis, helped fold laundry, held babies, and generally tried to fit into their routines during the interview rather than make them fit mine. These efforts helped to gather information in a less hierarchical way. It is important to remember, however, that the interview process has limitations in capturing the flow of social life.

2. Duff and Hollingshead (1968) in a study of medical care found that high percentages of the patients in both medical and surgical services received incorrect diagnoses. They attribute these high figures, in part, to the insulation of doctors from patients' concerns, leading to ignorance of crucial psychosocial aspects of people's lives and health.

3. The treatment for amenorrhea is presently a point of conflict for gynecology. Current research has been finding that to give hormones (in the pill) to women with amenorrhea may temporarily solve the problem, but over the long term this treatment can aggravate the problem by overwhelming the pituitary gland, decreasing the chances of normal recovery.

4. Many women have at some time in their lives been given comprehensive birth control information, but this information needs to be reviewed with women whenever they are making choices. People listen selectively to lectures and other sources. Thus in my interviews with women, often even women who reported having listened to in-depth discussions of all birth control methods in the past showed confusion about one or another method.

5. Barbara Seaman (1969, 1980) lists potential problems with the birth control pill in the chapter titles of her book: "Bloodclotting: No. 1 Danger; Strokes and the Pill; Heart Disease and the Pill; How the Pill Can Spoil Sex; Sterility and the Pill; Diabetes and the Pill; Genetic Changes and the Pill; The Pill and Jaundice, Thyroid Function, Weight Gain, Urinary Infections, Arthritis, Skin and Gum Problems; Depression and the Pill; Irritability and the Pill."

Dr. Harold Speert, a gynecologist at Columbia University, discusses the danger of the hormones in the birth control pill: "There is almost no organ or tissue which if studied has not been shown to be affected by the pill to some degree. . . . What troubles me is that the pill acts through the pituitary gland. The pituitary has been called 'the master gland.' . . . It does a lot of important things which shouldn't be interfered with. It's unrealistic to think that long-range effects will not be inevitable" (in Seaman 1969:25). Research on the possible effects of the pill continue to surface, such as in the study by Sloan et al. (1981), which details the connections between pill users and cardiovascular problems even up to nine years after stopping the pill. There has been recent information that the pill decreases pelvic inflammatory disease (PID), but once again this (like the research that the pill reduces risk of ovarian cancer) is controversial. For example, there is also recent research that links the pill to chlamydia, which in turn increases risk of PID. What we are left with are some *known* risks and many unanswered questions.

Although there is a wide range of opinions in the medical community on the safety and dangers of oral contraception, there is less controversy over the harmful effects of the IUD. All of the doctors in my study disapproved of this device, and despite its continued use in the population, they felt there was a general gynecological trend away from this method. Today, the IUD has largely been withdrawn from the market by manufacturers in the wake of the Dalkon Shield lawsuits, but a new copper IUD is being considered.

Interestingly, the staff members as well as their spouses in my data who did use birth control did not use the pill or the IUD. They chose the less risky barrier methods or sterilization, yet they most often suggested the pill to patients. This small sample is reflected in a report on Planned Parenthood workers. Oliva and Cobble conducted a survey of volunteers and staff at Planned Parenthood in the western states. Their findings showed that the majority of their 823-member sample used barrier methods or sterilization for prevention of pregnancy. Only 14.6 percent of the workers used the birth control pill in contrast to 70 percent of the client population (in Jacobs 1978).

6. The medical profession has always maintained that the risks from pregnancy are higher than the risks from the pill. These are problematic statistics in two ways. First, dangers from the pill are still in the experimental stage with the final tally not yet in. Second, statistical bookkeeping on this issue is difficult. When complications arise on the delivery table or during pregnancy, doctors generally feel confident recording them as childbirth-related. But when a woman goes into the hospital with a uterine infection and an IUD, doctors are often reticent to label any causal connection. Similarly, with the pill, when a stroke or a heart attack is tallied demographically it may show up in higher percentiles in pill users. At the individual level, however, doctors sometimes report strokes as strokes and heart attacks as heart attacks, in some cases failing even to report the use of the pill or IUD. Although doctors often report that they do think there is a causality that would explain the changes in demographic statistics, they also do not want explicitly to make such a connection because of what is claimed to be a lack of concrete scientific proof. Higher risk of liability for the doctor, the hospital, and the drug company could result if such connections are made explicit in individual cases.

5 | Good Doctors in a Bad Model

The question of immediate importance, from the sociological point of view, is why doctor-patient encounters such as those discussed in Chapter 4 are so systematically repeated. What is the source of the ideological attachment to such a notion as the fragmented person, separate from social life? How is such a system held together? How is it legitimized? Why is it that sincere doctors and conscientious patients adhere to such a narrow model? Why are women so easily silenced, and why do they allow entire life experiences and biographies to be erased from consideration? And finally, why do doctors, with the best of intentions, efface these social concerns in the first place?

Sexism and elitism are part of the answer and help clarify many of the examples given. The literature reviewed earlier systematically outlined the power embodied in modern medicine—the power to dominate attitudes toward the body and its ills and the incorporation of cultural assumptions toward women's roles in society. Power and patriarchal values are certainly involved, but a description of oppressive and exploitive aspects of the encounter does not explain or legitimize the structure of these doctor-patient interactions. Rather, these questions require an understanding of the ways in which cultural influences and ideological commitments weave throughout and shape our actions, whether we are aware of them or not, whether we understand them or not. In this case examination of the epistemological underpinnings of the scientific world view and its pervasiveness in social and individual assumptions is helpful.

There are, of course, important variations in the sciences. Basic research differs from clinical research, and applied science differs from research science. Clinical doctors, though perhaps engaging in various researches, are considered applied scientists. Despite enormous variety, there is what has come to be called a "scientific world view," a cultural layer of assumptions that influences all of modern society (see Harding 1986, Keller 1985, and Martin 1987 for discussion of a scientific epistemology). Such assumptions are subtle, but they are neither so elusive as to be incomprehensible nor so pervasive as to go unchallenged. In fact, it becomes crucial to make the abstract world view that surrounds us more visible to comprehend better and challenge the interactions discussed above.

SCIENCE AS A WORLD VIEW

> An interesting characteristic of a world view . . . is that the values located within it are so deep and so dear to us that we find it hard to imagine that we even have a "world view"—to us it is just reality—or that anyone else could not share it. By definition, those areas covered by a "world view" are those parts of life we take for granted, never questioning, and cannot envision decent, moral people not sharing. (Luker 1984:158)

In the above quotation, Kristin Luker is discussing the persuasive nature of the differing world views underlying the pro-life and pro-choice sides of the abortion debate. In a similar way doctors and patients bring to their meetings with each other unexamined, deeply entrenched assumptions about the world and therefore about medical care. Understanding these assumptions is somewhat more complicated than understanding the world views described by Luker. For Luker pro-life and pro-choice groups, despite being socialized in the same culture, are characterized by their differences. These groups are locked in political battle, and their daily lives are quite separate. Rarely do they find themselves in face-to-face interactions requiring a mutual decision. In fact, the abortion debate is characterized by the inability of its participants to reach mutual decisions. Not so for doctors and patients. Again, both are socialized in the same dominant culture, and at one level they share a world view about medicine in which doctors with their medical knowledge and technical skill are seen as the experts. Women bring their medical complaints to doctors, expecting the advances of modern science to be used to effect treatment. Doctors encourage and share this world view. In general, both have accepted the medical model as correct. Yet, while at one level there is a shared world view, at another doctors and patients bring to the medical relationship different assumptions about the world and about medical care. On one hand, doctors bring all their training, embedded in the social context of scientific and technical expertise, and apply it to problems of the body. Ideally they expect people to appreciate their knowledge, follow their instructions, and behave as good patients should. Women, on the other hand, bring their health concerns in a social matrix of family, work, finances, and so forth. Their health concerns are not strictly medical. They need doctors to hear these concerns and to extend and apply their knowledge accordingly. So as doctors and patients face each other in the examining room and prepare to reach mutual decisions, they do so in a context of overlapping and dissimilar world views.

In the last chapter this process was highlighted when the medical discourse was expanded with contextual discourse from the women's life experiences to show misunderstanding in medical interactions. Using the same technique here, understanding is sought. Once again expansions are used, but in this case they are examined to disclose the subtler discourse of a scientific world view. A close look at this discourse expands our understanding of the health care system and the treatment of women. Grasping the relationship among science, medicine, and gender provides a missing piece in the conceptual puzzle I have been discussing.

I am arguing for the inclusion of a scientific cosmology as one part of an open-ended, multifaceted explanation. I am not suggesting a simplistic causal analysis. In placing this facet (science) under the microscope, we can begin to see how the modern scientific explanatory system conceptually influences our views of human beings and society as it influences medical theory. This vision contributes to our understanding of the conflict between doctors' biomedical conceptions and people's more contextual understandings. An examination of the scientific metaphor of the body as machine with an emphasis on the specific etiology of disease, separate from the conscious mind and social life, under the care of a scientific expert, provides a conceptual level from which to help understand the doctor-patient relationship. Concomitantly with the scientific revolution, separations between emotions and reason were reformulated with the former being seen as feminine and the latter masculine. These conceptualizations have had an important influence on the doctor-patient relationship, especially when the patient is a woman—points I will discuss later in this chapter.

A main theme of this book has been that health care is a relationship in which the participants can be observed in concert and their communication analyzed. To limit the analyses to the doctor-patient relationship insulated from larger contexts, however, would be to make the same mistake doctors make when they treat patients separated from their social lives. Starting at the core of medicine—the communication between doctor and patient—we can move out, layer by layer, to analyze the way science influences this relationship, developing a larger picture in the process.

Like other world views, science, once established, becomes largely invisible. What in fact has a long historical, social development is assumed and taken for granted. To connect the scientific world view with the doctor-patient relationship, it first becomes necessary to outline socially constructed aspects of science and then to explore the use of science as an explanatory theory in modern societies. For it is this progression that sets the stage to consider how the image of women and the cultural authority of doctors are entwined with a scientific cosmology.

THE SOCIAL CONSTRUCTION OF SCIENCE

One of the problems for the study of science as a social construction is the prevailing view in modern society that it is not socially constructed. In a senior seminar in critical health issues, I opened the class with a question: What is the prevailing world view in our society today? Many answers were given; none was correct. When I told this story to a wide variety of colleagues expecting shared amazement at the students' confusion, I received equally surprising responses. As Luker states, the world views so deeply embedded in our society and consciousness go largely unnoticed. The scientific world view is accepted by scientists and laypeople alike. It is a belief system that denies its own reality as a world view, believing instead that it is a series of truths about knowing and controlling the unpredictable world we live in.

As scholars have shown in detail, modern science and the conceptual shifts that came with it arose at a particular moment in history and were embedded in complex social contexts. Robert Merton's statement about the development of the Protestant ethic is equally relevant here: "[Such changes are] at once a direct expression of dominant values and an independent source of new motivation" (1973:228). Over time the development of scientific thought has had an enormous impact on our ways of knowing and seeing, not the least of which is our confusion that such a world view even exists.

Carolyn Merchant (1980), Hilary and Steven Rose (1969), and Robert Merton (1973) tie the rise of the scientific revolution to sweeping social and economic changes that include increasing urbanization, wider trade, and the rise of Protestantism. Merchant describes these changes in ecological terms. By integrating nature and culture in her analysis, she explores the peasant-landlord relationship to natural resources and sees capitalist control centered on profit. The organic, holistic model—living with nature to survive—changed to a mechanistic model of exploiting nature for the benefit of a few. In this new belief system, people and nature were exploited for profit. Mother Nature, once seen as vital and giving, became something that could be broken down into atomistic parts to be understood, controlled, and used to man's advantage. As the new symbolic system redefined nature, the view of women changed as well. Both were wayward, unpredictable, and in need of control. Merchant's analysis in *The Death of Nature* includes the death of women—the rendering of the feminine as passive and, I would add, in need of expert attention.

Just as Max Weber tied industrious Puritan sentiments to economic change (to capitalism), Merton describes the rise of modern science as associated with religion, the Protestant Reformation. He argues that Puritan sentiments and beliefs "build a new bridge between the transcendental and human action, thus supplying a motive force for the new science" (1973:229). Merton suggests that this bourgeois rationality was conducive to the rise of science and technology.

For each of these social theorists the scientific revolution took place at a historical crossroads, creating a break between science and religion and a change from a feudal to a capitalist society. Both a scientific world view and capitalism were entwined with and dependent on a further conceptual shift—the rise of individualism. Just as Galileo, astronomer and mathematician, had divided the natural world into individual particles in constant motion, Hobbes, mathematician and social thinker, defined people as individual, autonomous units. Edgar Zilsel points out, "In medieval society the individual was bound to the traditions of the group to which he [sic] unalterably belonged. In early capitalism economic success depended on the spirit of enterprise of the individual" (1974:80). The atomistic structure observable in the purely intellectual pursuits of Galileo's vision of the universe and Hobbes's social order fit perfectly with these social changes. Industrialization required a new kind of labor different from that of the feudal order. Peasants connected to the land and tradition were to be transformed into autonomous workers in the factory run by autonomous entrepreneurs separated from traditions and any social responsibilities except to yield profit. People defined as disparate individuals became as interchangeable as machine parts in the interests of the new capitalist classes.

The developing social order thus required both a new definition of nature and a new definition of people. People had dominion over nature, but in this regard not all people were equal. Masculine dominance of female nature was a metaphor for men to control women and the environment; however, it only applied to some men. The ideological commitment to dominance was reflected in class and gender divisions that complemented capitalism with workers of both sexes, providing a valuable resource. Thus the rise of scientific explanations legitimized the new approach to people and to labor as well as to nature.

None of these writers suggests simple, causal arguments about science and its growth; rather, each attempts to place science in context. Without this context it is impossible to understand the way we live and think in the modern world. Even with this context what we see are changes both gradual and rapid. Historically, these changes were reflected in as well as accredited to a small number of relatively disparate scientific philosophers of the seventeenth century. These philosophers were not professionals working within an organized, bureaucratically funded institution. Such thinkers as Copernicus (connected to the church), Newton (the university), Galileo, Brahe, and Kepler (grants from royalty), Boyle and Bacon (independent means), and Harvey (physician) (Rose and Rose 1969:9) did their own work, often were amateurs, and received their funds from a variety of nonbureaucratic sources. The scientific enterprise as we know it was in its infancy. It grew to become, by the nineteenth century, an accepted, entrenched, and sophisticated social reality. The institutionalization of science brought with it the institutionalization of the expert to find the facts and translate them to the rest of society. Just as religious leaders told the people what God wanted, scientists could tell people what the world was all about—whether it be what the earth was made of to facilitate mining or the relationship between skull size and intelligence to understand hierarchy of race and gender.

The expert most important for this book is the physician—an applied scientist. Doctors, having been around for centuries, were able to claim a new cultural authority based on their supposed scientific expertise. Just as priests conducted intercessionary prayer to care for their followers, doctors could now practice interventionary medicine to cure their patients. The scientist, rather than the priest, slowly became the authorized expert who possessed the knowledge to explain the world or, with medical science, to explain and treat the body. Scientists became the new truthsayers, and just as the public had taken its cues from the church it now took them from science. Religion required faith. Medicine required trust.

SCIENCE AS SOCIAL THEORY

Perhaps the clearest way to begin to talk about science as a social theory is to look at the concept of progress. Today we define progress as the accumulation of knowledge (primarily scientific knowledge) and its application through technological advances. To describe a way of thinking as nonprogressive is pejorative, but this understanding is fairly new. In the Middle Ages progress was not in favor. To work toward change or inquire into existence and the status of the world was to question God's order. To think "progressively" was to overstep the bounds of being human by taking on God's task. Thus such a seemingly simple concept as progress, one that we assume to be universally good, is in fact historically and culturally specific. I am arguing here that it is part of a social theory that defines for us what our society values.

In this conception of science, scientists are seen as the movers and shakers; we the public are the recipients. Funding may come from specific interest groups such as industry or government, but these groups are seen as having no influence on the autonomy and integrity of science. The scientific method of fact-finding, based on a commitment to objectivity, undergirds a vision of science in America as so justifiably autonomous that regulation is largely entrusted to scientists themselves.[1] It is generally accepted that scientists do their work detached from future use and responsibility—finding the facts that others in society may use or abuse.

Once again my point is that this way of seeing presents a social theory that separates scientific facts or truths from the social context in which they arise and are used—that negates its own participation in the social construction of a scientific world view.

The epistemological underpinnings of this way of seeing are rooted in a vision of pure, objective inquiry in which observed facts confirm or disconfirm hypotheses. Once a hypothesis has been tested repeatedly and confirmed, it becomes a law, a statement of universal fact. Such a statement does not tell us why certain things happen but that they do. Although at first glance these statements may appear static, William Broad and Nicholas Wade point out that "an important feature of the structure [of science] is its flexibility" (1982:17) to revise laws by gathering new scientific facts. Empirical testing of validity or falsification supports the claim of objectively justifiable knowledge. The flexibility of this process lies in the ideal of accumulating truth by trial and retrial. The scientific revolution and the growth of the ideals of rationality make it possible to criticize the very system they support. Skepticism and questioning are integral to the scientific enterprise. The inflexibility lies in a commitment to an external reality that is discoverable cumulatively through the application of objective methods. Historical connections and human influences are not considered part of science. Any connection between descriptions of the world and human assumptions or between categories and categorizers is denied. Rather, science is seen as value-free, requiring skepticism at all levels, with a knowledge base said to consist of not yet disproved hypotheses and proven laws. This version of reality defines scientific method as *the* approach to understanding the world. It is a system based on quantifiable, objective facts separate from social or contextual life and nature separate from society. In this century the collection of facts by neutral, value-free scientists to prove truths about the world we live in has itself become a taken-for-granted scientific fact—a fact scientists in their daily work are, for the most part, rarely aware of.

The scientist Stephen Jay Gould is one of a growing number of people to question these "unquestionable" facts of science (see Knorr-Cetina 1981 for detailed discussion of the contextual nature of science). He joins others in emphasizing that science is a value-laden enterprise: "I believe that science must be understood as a social phenomenon, a gutsy human enterprise, not the work of robots programmed to collect pure information" (1981:21). To suppose that pure scientific thought and research can be separable from historical and social consideration is increasingly seen as a flawed theory. Gould is joined by others questioning the cultural definitions of science as an objective fact-finding mission aimed at understanding and controlling wayward nature (with nature representing and being represented by the feminine). Ruth Bleier has pointed out, "Science is *not* the neutral, dispassionate, value-free pursuit of Truth; . . . scientists are not objective, disinterested, or culturally disengaged from the questions they ask of nature or the methods they use to frame their answers" (1984: 193). And Margaret Osler argues, "The history of science teaches us that the choice of assumptions and of methods as well as the choice of questions to be investigated are choices based on values" (in Bleier 1984:4). Bleier argues further that the method used and the interpretation of results that follows can be manipulated, usually unintentionally, in accordance with a researcher's assumptions. The argument being made here supports the claim that scientific theory is a social theory: science is connected to social values and interests, scientific questions are asked within a social context, and the scientific method, supposed to provide protection against individual researchers' biases, is equally contextually embedded. In other words, scientific theories, methods, and interpretations are social activities tied to historical periods and particular cultural and individual expectations and values.[2]

Despite these criticisms, there is no conspiracy in science. Rather, a neutral, value-free cloak becomes a wrap of mystification which often encloses the imaginations of scientists as well as the general public. Further, such critiques of science by no means claim that science cannot contribute to knowledge. Technology is an often-cited example of scientific success. Clearly technological innovations frequently work whether based on scientific discoveries or not. That is, they produce results. The question being addressed, however, is not whether the scientific enterprise works. The central questions are how science functions as a social theory and whether it should hold the privileged position that it does, affecting everyone in society—a position based on the assumption that it is somehow pure, interest-free, and untainted.

The answers to these questions are not without consequences. The Brighton Women and Science Group (1980) argues that our blind faith in scientific objectivity "and its practice, the disinterested pursuit of truth" has "in the service of Capitalist production and imperialist expansion given us the atom bomb, the neutron bomb, and nuclear reactors. . . . In the service of social control science has offered us theories of innate differences between people." As I argue elsewhere, it also contributes to the cultural authority of doctors and to the diseasing of women and their bodies (Todd 1983).

The scientific ethos heavily flavors all scientific and medical inquiry. The scientific equation that influences all disciplines delivers a certain knowledge that limits our ability to construct other forms of inquiry. The academic disciplines are segmented into little pieces. Just as medicine has conceptualized the body in parts or organs separated from contextual concerns, scholarship is narrowly defined. For example, we often assume separations called for in a scientific cosmology. Facts are seen as separate from values, morality and ethics as separate from scientific truths. Social sciences, shaped under the shadow of the natural sciences, seek the hard, factual truths about society in as objective a manner as possible. Moral questions such as, What is a good society? What makes for the best society and for whom? How can equity be promoted? How can science and technology help us to reach these goals? tend to be left to the ethicists—put off in a little compartment with yet another expert. Since morality is seen as "soft," "subjective," and "unscientific," the moral questions receive low priority; there are no universals to be plumbed here. It is important to remember that it is within the social theory of scientific reasoning that these questions can be so ignored; that the choice *not* to ask them *is* an unacknowledged moral choice.

An understanding of the rise of a scientific world view as social theory frames the dynamics between doctors and patients discussed in earlier chapters. Modern science as a model of inquiry strongly influenced contemporary medical theory and practice. Although the connections between practical scientific research and medical knowledge are well recognized, less obvious are the influences on health care of the broader scientific attitudes toward the body/nature, mind/society, and female/feminine. The literature reviewed and the data discussed thus far highlight women's medical treatment for reproductive concerns. Women find themselves in an unequal relationship in which their knowledge and interpretations are often disregarded; their bodies are fragmented and treated as objectifiable parts separate from the rest of their lives. Women, competent outside of the doctors' offices, once inside were treated as incompetent. They seemingly accepted this definition. In these repeated scenarios the discourse of science is juxtaposed and entwined with the discourse of medical practice and a discourse of gender.

WOMEN AND SCIENCE

Elizabeth Fee asks the question, "Is there a conflict of interest between women's values and the values of science?" (1983:9). She then goes on to argue that within the scientific framework, the question makes little sense since dominant interpretations of science lay no claim to values. From a feminist perspective, however, the question makes a great deal of sense. In recent years a growing body of scholarship has asserted that indeed science is value-oriented and this orientation is, among others, a masculine one.

The scientific process has had additional consequences for women. The assumptions of hierarchy and dominance as natural in nature and society have been used "scientifically" to reinforce a view of women as inferior. Modern medicine is a good example. Defined as the scientific and thus solely credible source of knowledge on health, disease, and reproduction, medicine has both reflected and reinforced this definition of women. Medical practitioners translate abstract scientific assumptions about gender into daily realities for women in terms of their bodies. As it reflects and reinforces the image of women as inferior, the practice of medicine is one among many possible forms of social control. It contributes to women's status (or lack thereof) as it reinforces the scientific cosmology.

The questions can be asked, weren't women considered inferior long before the rise of modern science and the practice of modern medicine? Were not hierarchy and domination parts of the social fabric before the scientific revolution? Yes, of course; but the scientific age lends its authority to these views, making them facts—irrefutable based on their biological origins, unchangeable because rooted in nature, applicable to all women. A long tradition of sexual inequality has been made scientifically true.

Anthropologists have long pointed out the following oppositional, binary categories that exist in many societies whether pre- or post-scientific and industrial revolutions:

nature	versus	culture
wild	versus	tame
raw	versus	cooked
child	versus	adult
female	versus	male

Categories take on a more political tone in the following divisions:

colonizer	versus	colonized
proletarian	versus	capitalist
female	versus	male

A further categorization adds an emphatic grounding in modern industrial and scientific conceptualizations:

nature	versus	culture
body	versus	mind
subjectivity	versus	objectivity
private realm	versus	public realm
feeling	versus	thinking
reproducers	versus	producers
emotional woman	versus	rational man

In this latter categorization women become defined as the feeling, emotional reproducers, caring for the family and home, and representing "Mother" nature. Both women and nature reproduce the world—give birth—and in so doing are seen as needing to be controlled, their power potentially dangerous and unpredictable. Men are seen as the rational thinkers producing in the workplace and objectively controlling nature and women—making the mysterious knowable and controllable. The world becomes a polarity between the generic masculine and the generic feminine, each gender heavily laden with a set of scientifically determined qualities. The message is that the sociohistorical development of property and gender relations are really "natural" developments (MacCormack 1980:20). This polarity is put forth and assumed as value-free scientific fact and universal truth.

The importance of these gender distinctions lies in the new definition of woman and all that is feminine. The world is divided into the knower (scientist, mind, masculine) and the knowable (nature, body, feminine). The decks are stacked, the rules of the game set, with the players separated and distanced from each other. The knower uses reason to dominate the knowable; feelings and emotions give way to objective observation. For women this is a losing game: "In this process, the characterization of both the scientific mind and its modes of access to knowledge as masculine is indeed significant. Masculine here connotes, as it so often does, autonomy, separation, and distance. It connotes a radical rejection of any commingling of subject and object, which are, it now appears, quite consistently identified as male and female" (Keller 1983:191). Evelyn Fox Keller goes on to explore the masculine stance science takes as it "conquers" and "masters" nature. She asserts that the masculinity of science leads to the majority of scientists being men, not the other way around. The origins are in belief not in reality—in a world view that informs reality and in turn is strengthened by that reality.

This masculinist bias is reflected in all stages of scientific research, from the selection of scientists and their access to facilities, to the choice of research topics, experimental subjects, and methods of observation, to the interpretation of data and data analysis, to the final publication of results and the popularization of those results by the press. At each stage this bias works against women (Messing 1983:76). Karen Messing goes on to point out that "scientists, protected by their image as zealous seekers after truth, have been allowed to say the most outrageous things about women with impunity" (p. 84).

Scholars from varying theoretical perspectives have provided an array of accounts to explain "the woman question." First, male dominance is "natural," beyond social or human tinkering—man-the-hunter theories and sociobiology. Women and men should play out their naturally prescribed roles maintaining the social order, which "objectively" defines women as inferior and then uses these definitions to keep women in inferior positions. There is a caveat, however, to explain the success of some women. They do not defy their biological destiny. Some women become scientists, doctors, *and* mothers without challenging the existing order or assumptions. They simply are seen as men in the workplace and women in the home.

A second view denies the differences (except anatomical) between men and women. These differences between the sexes, it is claimed, are a pretext to exclude women from production, keeping them reproducing and in the home. This position calls for equality of opportunity for both the sexes and an end to discrimination. Women can do what men can do and should be allowed their piece of the pie. The shape of the pie remains undisputed.

A third position is more challenging. The differences between the masculine and feminine worlds are acknowledged, although seen as rooted in historical time and place rather than purely in nature. The feminine characterizations of emotion, feeling, and subjectivity are reconceptualized and promoted from their inferior position to one of equal respect. Elevating the feminine carries the potential of enlightenment for science and society. For example, Jean Baker Miller (1976) criticizes the masculine ideals as stunted in caring and emotional growth—qualities crucial to a good society. The world would be a better place if feminine strengths were reevaluated and incorporated into the place of importance they deserve. It is not enough to give women equal opportunity in a problematic system; the system itself must change: "The problem . . . is located not in women, but in the particular character of our production of scientific knowledge. In this view, the problem is not one of making women more scientific, but of making science less masculine. When masculinity is seen as an incomplete and thus distorted form of humanity, the issue of making science and technology less masculine is also the issue of making it more completely human" (Fee 1983:15).

Implicit in the perspectives discussed so far is an essentialist view of women: (1) women are not men and are therefore inferior; (2) if equal opportunity is provided for women, this will lead to change; (3) if the ideology is reshaped, women will benefit. In each case, women, by implication all women, are lumped together. Missing in many of these critiques is an analysis of differences among women in race, class, ethnicity, sexual identity, able-bodiedness, and lived experience. It is just this concern for difference that is addressed by deconstructionists. They argue that binary categories as laid out above confer symmetry or declare opposition in a fictitious manner. By this I take them to mean that although there are differences, for example, between men and women or among men and among women, these differences are neither major enough to constitute the social uses of binary oppositions—masculine versus feminine—nor unitary symmetries—man or woman. The project for deconstructionists is to unravel these binary oppositions by revealing the discontinuities in what are typically seen as "unified texts," or for my purposes, belief systems.[3]

These discussions of how to understand women's place present us with a challenge—how to throw out the bathwater but keep the baby. Masculine and feminine traits must be kept in historical perspective lest we go from one extreme to the other, risking a new form of biological determinism: the feminine as universal and, at least by implication, better. Donna Harraway raises the disturbing dilemma that if "all scientific statements are historical fictions made facts through the exercise of power [there will be] trouble when feminists want to talk about producing *feminist* science which is more *true*" (1981:478). In other words, if the one is socially constructed and value-laden, how can the replacement be value-neutral fact, when such concepts as value-neutral have been defined as unreal and masculinist? This is a dilemma that will take many minds much work to unravel. Perhaps for our purposes here, emphasis on the dual roles of women's experiences and historical social contexts, entwined as they are, can reshape the problem (deleting the idea of "fictions" altogether), offering some insights.

For example, in the last chapter women's experiences are important starting places for a deeper understanding of health care even if these experiences are not immediately grasped by the participants: "Those who construct the standpoint of women must begin from women's experience as women describe it, but they must go beyond that experience theoretically and ultimately may require that women's experience be redescribed" (Jaggar 1983 : 384).

People's experiences, though socially grounded and influenced, begin to tell us much about any historical moment. Alison Jaggar continues,

> The concept of women's standpoint is not theory-neutral. Like every episte-
> mology, it is conceptually linked to a certain ontology: its model of how knowl-
> edge is achieved necessarily presupposes certain general features of human
> nature and human social life. Whether or not one accepts socialist feminist
> epistemology thus depends in part on whether or not one accepts the general
> view of reality on which it rests. . . . It also offers [through unraveling domi-
> nant male biases] at least a method for discovering the material reasons for its
> own emergence in this particular historical period. (p. 385)

The challenge is to begin to understand the role that science has played as a social theory in constructing women's place. On the basis of this understanding we will be better able to construct new definitions of masculinity and femininity that do not imply new facts but rather a new equity.

This challenge does not encourage an antiscientific, antitechnology pessimism leading to a romantic, back-to-nature view. In this century, particularly since World War II, the rationality of science which allows for self-criticism has been replaced by a romanticism of its own. This romanticism is all too often devoid of the necessary criticism that is part and parcel of science and must be viewed with a skeptical eye. Both rationality and emotion are necessary. Rationality allows for some level of objectivity to prevail over a totally subjective perception, and this is important in society for men and women. The realm of reason is uniquely developed in human beings, monkeys who can type notwithstanding, but so are feelings and emotions. Barbara McClintock, the Nobel Prize–winning geneticist, as described by Keller in her book appropriately entitled *A Feeling for the Organism* (1983), details the entwining of an emotional and rational approach to scientific inquiry with innovative results. The model she describes is a holistic, intuitive one that does not sacrifice the use of reason. At the level of social theory, a growing discussion addresses how to rethink a scientific world view, trying to hold onto what is enlightening and dispense with what is oppressive (see Wright, in progress). At the level of scientific theory, however, despite argument to the contrary, the assumptions that nature and the feminine need to be tamed remain entrenched. Modern medicine, as applied science, has historically played a major role in translating these assumptions into concrete medical practices that have major consequences for women's lives. A brief discussion of the scientific revolution and the birth of modern medicine will further explicate these connections.

THE SCIENTIFIC REVOLUTION AND MODERN MEDICINE

> We can employ these entities physiological laws for all the purposes for which they are suited, and so make ourselves masters and possessors of nature. This would not only be desirable in bringing about the invention of an infinity of devices to enable us to enjoy the fruits of agriculture and all the wealth of the each without labor, but even more so in conserving health. (Descartes 1960:45–46)

René Descartes's philosophical separation of the mind from the body became a reference, and justification, for the application of the new scientific principles to the realm of health and medicine. The body became subject to an understanding based on the study of its own internal mechanisms, biological processes which worked universally and independently of the conscious mind. The mind preserved the unique human ability to reason; the body was pure matter. Descartes, an admirer of Harvey, went beyond the hydraulics of blood to the hydraulics of the body—a body that could be conceptualized and treated as a machine.

Thomas McKeown explicates the mind-body dualism in his study of the contributions of scientific ideology to theories of health. He discusses the two competing concepts of health articulated philosophically in the seventeenth century: (1) health preserved by way of life and (2) health restored by treatment of disease: "Philosophically the seventeenth century was a turning point in the balance between the two concepts. Galileo has shown that scientific methods were capable of providing a mechanical interpretation of the physical world, and Descartes saw no reason why the same principles should not be extended to living things. He conceived of the body as a machine, governed entirely by the laws of physics, which might be taken apart and reassembled if its structure and function were fully understood" (1976:2).

The alchemists had envisioned holism—mind, spirit, and body, as well as connections between masculine and feminine. The new men of science envisioned separations and reductions. The seventeenth century has had an enormous impact on how we think about matters of medicine and disease. It was not until the nineteenth century, however, that these thoughts began to influence practice. Certainly changes in medical practice were a continuous process, but it was in the nineteenth century that medical men became members of a consolidated profession, systematically developing and practicing scientific medicine. Stanley Reiser (1978) argues that the production of new medical technologies in the nineteenth and twentieth centuries changed the medical encounter from a subjective, person-centered focus to a more objective, mechanistic one, dependent on technological devices and mechanistic definitions. Changes in attitudes toward the body and the growth of medical technology combined to reorganize medical care.

From the Middle Ages to the late eighteenth century, doctors understood disease from (1) the patients' statements regarding their illnesses and (2) the doctors' sensory observations of the signs of illness and demeanor of the patient. People were active participants in the interaction, which often took place in the patient's home (Reiser 1978). Although treatment was technically unsophisticated and sometimes dangerous, it centered around people's concerns and satisfaction. Throughout the nineteenth century increased urbanization and industrialization heralded in hospitals' fulfilling the need for large centers to treat the mass of urban poor and sick. The patient began to lose center stage as people's accounts were replaced by technologically based diagnoses, an emphasis on statistical data, and disease classifications. Becoming increasingly sophisticated, modern medicine increasingly emphasized intervention. First, the stethoscope introduced diagnosis based on the pathology of sound. The doctor could hear these sounds, the patient could not, initiating a withdrawal of the doctor from the person-centered signs of illness. Distancing trends continued with the invention of the ophthalmoscope, laryngoscope, x-ray, and microscope. The x-ray and microscope allowed group evaluation of people without their even being present. Developments such as these estranged doctors from trust in empirical understandings of people and their illnesses. By the late nineteenth century and twentieth century this trend toward "objectivity" increased with the use of numerical graphs to record bodily symptoms (Reiser 1978). A mechanistic approach to the body (as well as to nature) prevailed, and more holistic practices such as vitalism suffered defeat.

The rise of commercial laboratories and large centralized medical complexes, along with the increasing use of the computer to process medical data and perform diagnoses, have provided the finishing touches to laboratory medicine. These technologies are used to increase medicine's "scientific" legitimacy, and doctors' dependence on people to effect a cure decreases—the ill become, even more, the hosts for organs and bacteria. A recent advertisement for video consoles at a nurses' station heralded further distance between patients and practitioners. The ad featured a doctor and nurse observing a panorama of patients on video screens. Technical observational opportunity combined with personal attention has much to offer patient care. The caption of this ad, however, had something else in mind, implying that the practitioner might never have to touch another patient. Computerization, for example, may be an invaluable and essential tool for medical care, with each technological advance offering some benefit. The costs, however, need to be understood.

Today medicine has refined a mechanistic definition of the body which first fragmented the patient into parts and later into cells. This view has encouraged such medical advances as new technologies, vaccinations, anesthesia, antibiotics, and so forth, but it has also, as Reiser details, led to greater distance between doctors and patients. In "a shift from a person-oriented to an object-oriented cosmology," the patient lost the status of person. Patients, the subjects of medicine, concomitantly became its objects. Doctors became a consolidated profession, legitimized in part (as time went on) by their association with science. Science provided the world view, the tools, and the stance—active investigator, passive investigated. Just as scientists separated themselves from nature, doctors separated themselves from their patients.

The mind conceptualized as separate from the body, doctors distanced from the people they served, and individuals reduced to machine parts understood through universal laws are separations that leave human beings and their role in the universe in an interesting position. In the new physics God is redefined as a part-time mechanic. The new objective, machinelike world based on universal laws can be understood only by human reason and the ability to experiment. Enter the scientist and the scientific doctor. Nature is based on universal laws, but only a few can hope to uncover these laws. The rest of the population lives in a world where opinions need correction by dispassionate experts,[4] and scientists are the experts. Through careful education in the objective, mechanical realm, scientists use the power of reason to gain knowledge of underlying causation, to control nature and the universe. By similar methods the scientific doctor seeks control of the body. In the process people have been atomized, anatomized, and removed from the center of the universe. By the end of the nineteenth century, scientific medicine was entrenched and social or environmental causation or influence on disease for the most part excluded from medical attention.

> Conceptually, the image of the human body as a single, integrated organism—with effects on one part of the body having effects upon the rest of the body—was finally eliminated from the mainstream of medical thought. . . . Specialization under scientific medicine began to emphasize individual systems or organs to the exclusion of the totality of the body. . . . The accumulation of knowledge in medicine (i.e., research) was also drastically influenced by the new paradigm. By definition, scientific medicine rejected the idea of social causality of disease or illness since the social basis of humanity was placed out-

side the realm of what was considered scientific. Research was structured in such a way as to reinforce this exclusion of social causality. The predominant focus of medical research became pathology and pathological anatomy. Therapeutics, hygiene, and symptomatology, all mainstays of wholistic medicine, were largely ignored. (Berliner 1975:576–77)

Osherson and AmaraSingham sum up the evolution of the parameters of our current medical model originating from the seventeenth and eighteenth centuries:

> In the evolving emphasis on objective, physical measurement we can see the concern with defining disease as deviation from the normal or average; in the emphasis on underlying causation, not visible to the subjective senses but objectively rooted in the physical world, we find the roots of the search for generic, universal diseases [and causes]; and the high value placed on the dispassionate, objective investigator empirically observing the basic mechanisms of nature is an important source of the belief in the scientific neutrality of medicine. (1981:224–25)

These transformations evolved slowly. Overviews provide a sense of change; historical scholarship provides the details. Susan Bell's research is an example of such historical detail. She examines the relationship between laboratory science and clinical medicine in the development of DES (the synthetic estrogen diethylstilbestrol) in the late 1930s and early 1940s. Scientific discoveries of hormonal development in the female cycle established menopause as a normal, physiological part of women's lives as opposed to earlier "crisis" definitions. At the same time, the focus on hormones pared the topic of inquiry to specific biological processes and to hormonal deficiencies, excluding psychosocial and environmental influences. In one breath menopause became defined as a part of all women's physiological lives, and in the next it was seen as a deficiency disease in need of medical management. Clinical doctors were both drawn to and skeptical of the laboratory research on DES and menopause. Some doctors, though excited by the possibilities of keener, generalizable scientific precision, also warned that sensitivity to individuals was important. Generalizability and detail conflicted, and "they neither rejected nor embraced laboratory science wholeheartedly" (Bell 1984:31). The clinicians' talents at this time were increasingly taking second place to the avalanche of new scientific findings relevant to health care. One suspects that an element of power and prestige is involved. Doctors wanted to incorporate the fruits of laboratory science into their practices while holding onto their own clinical contributions. Probably they also wanted to deliver the best possible health care holding onto personal relationships with patients and not wanting all of their success attributed to remote, generalizable research. This history is characterized by competition as well as by an alliance between laboratory science and clinical medicine, characteristics that continue today.

> "It has seemed to me that clinicians are developing a sort of inferiority complex in the study of endocrine problems, so awed are they by the brilliant contributions which have been coming from the laboratory, and so dependent have they become upon the laboratory workers for the ammunition which they so sorely need in their own clinical work. . . . And yet there are certain advantages which the clinician enjoys over the laboratory worker." (Novak 1939: 432, in Bell 1984:5)

Medicine and science are intricately entwined. Today, modern medicine, resting heavily on the credentials and cultural status of science, takes as its primary concern the cure of disease (as opposed to, for example, the prevention of ill health) and approaches this task with a fundamental imagery of biological-physiological causality. Although not reducible to the early mechanical philosophy, this imagery envisions biochemical elements invading the body, elements which must be rooted out and countered with other biochemical agents to be cured. Even the body as a whole, the complex interrelatedness of its parts, is not included as a conceptual reality in medical imagery (Powles 1973). The metaphors are biological, deeply mechanistic, and internally complete. There is little room, if any, for other explanatory factors such as social life, state of mind, economic concerns, or cultural beliefs.

McKeown sums up these historical changes and their impact on medicine today and asks the question, Does modern medicine work?

> The approach to biology and medicine established in the seventeenth century was an engineering one based on a physical model; its consequences are even more conspicuous today, largely because the resources of the physical and chemical sciences are so much greater. Physics, chemistry, and biology are considered to be the sciences basic to medicine; medical education begins with study of the structure and function of the body, continues with examination of disease processes and ends with clinical instruction on selected sick people. Medical service is dominated by the image of the acute hospital where the technological resources are concentrated, and much less attention is given to environmental and behavioral determinants of disease. . . . The question, therefore, is not whether the engineering approach is predominant in medicine, which would hardly be disputed, but whether it is seriously deficient as a conceptualization of the problem of human health. (1976:6)

He goes on to argue that in fact the model is indeed deficient and asserts that "the modern improvement in health was initiated and carried quite a long way with little assistance from science and technology" (p. 9).

In other words, the value of scientific medicine itself has come under attack in recent years. Serious questions have been asked about the most successful techniques for the achievement of individual and social health. Historical claims of systematic contributions have been debunked, specifically the conquering of the killer diseases such as cholera, tuberculosis, and typhoid. In addition, the vaunted claims of the modern medical drugs and technologies have been seriously challenged. These questions by no means discredit all that science, medicine, and technology have to offer or deny the importance of antibiotics and such vaccines as the Salk polio vaccine. In fact, increased primary care programs, particularly when combined with environmental regulations and changes, have led to better health in America. As mentioned in Chapter 1, however, it has been some time since medical science has had a major breakthrough—one that affects the lives of a large proportion of the population. The major health problems of this age—cancer and more recently viruses such as herpes and AIDS—remain largely unchecked. Furthermore, the medical profession is limited by its own belief system, relying on it to the exclusion of alternative approaches, often overusing the advances offered. For example, the overprescription of antibiotics and the increasing resistance of bacteria to these drugs are growing problems. Modern scientific medicine thus can have serious consequences, even if it sometimes "works."[5]

Discussed above is the development of a medical model that has effects, in a general way, on our very conception of medical practice. McKeown asks and answers the question: "Is this model deficient for health care?" He answers that it is. I argue that such error embodies a misconception of illness and health, nature, and society. In sum, at the level of epistemology, a medical mistake has been made. Science as a social theory defines the social world and human nature and has been applied to health, illness, and the body. This theory is based on the ideal of objective truth and progress emanating from natural laws devoid of social, contextual concerns—a social theory that in essence denies the existence of its own social, contextual origins. If the scientific enterprise is a fact-finding mission in search of universal laws, truth is the logical outcome and human-social-cultural-historical concerns (such as power structures, class, race, or gender) are by definition denied. If scientific medicine is defined as objective facts, contextual knowledge is once again ignored. In either case one is left in the position of having to accept truth as it has been defined. You can't fight truth. This point is the hardest to grasp, the one that mystifies the most. For in order to fight, one has to know what one is fighting, but as a quotation early in this chapter states, one of the characteristics of a world view is its invisibility, its taken-for-granted character. The scientific world view remains for the most part elusive and intact. Once this view is located within a specific historical context and seen as socially created, the door is open for investigation, criticism, and potential revision.

I was struck as I analyzed the data in prior chapters with the power of the medical model, the way it functioned as a world view. Doctors were unaware that it existed. When faced with criticism of aspects of this model, the medical profession demonstrates resistance. Of particular interest here is the resistance to challenges that bring people's contextual lives into what are defined as biomedical topics. There is no awareness that biomedical topics are also contextual and that the very separation of the social and the biomedical is a social, historical development. It is necessary for the invisible to become visible and for us all to recognize that people's contextual knowledge not only is compatible with medical knowledge but is essential to the delivery of high-quality health care.

Science and the Doctor-Patient Relationship

What does all of this mean for the doctor-patient relationship and more specifically for the questions raised at the beginning of this chapter? Women in my study and the data discussed earlier were held to a narrow definition of their concerns. Women's social, biographical material was repeatedly truncated by doctors who wanted to focus on the medical matter at hand— the body, its control, and its treatment. The doctor-patient relationship is shaped by these dynamics, and medical interactions take on a new sense when examined in this light. Doctors, as dispassionate experts, objective practitioners, scientifically apply universal physical laws to the mechanical organ/body of the patient. This ideal type, of course, is formally laid out and unrealistic. Guesswork, unknowns, uncertainty, and so forth, are as much a part of medicine and science as any other part of life. The belief system is a powerful one, however. Doctors are seen as the knowers, patients the knowables. These factors can be seen in each of the three types of interactions discussed in Chapter 4.

Maria Martinez and Corinne Conrad represented a pattern in which women tried to insert information into the medical dialogue. Maria came to the doctor with a personal story to tell concerning her history and her fear of pain with the IUD, contextual information. The doctor, basing his knowledge on conventional medical wisdom, misunderstood. This misunderstanding was rooted in a lack of attention to women's experiences. Corinne similarly tried to insert contextual information. The doctor interrupted, designating such talk as inappropriate. Both women, sharing this world view, abbreviated themselves to accommodate the medical model. Both raised questions, and one can assume that the issues raised were important to them. These questions expressed the women's interpretations of their problems. Yet neither trusted her interpretation enough to challenge the doctors by insisting on her views. Neither Maria nor Corinne was allowed to tell her story completely; such contextual information is not generally considered medically relevant. And in the final analysis, each received inadequate care when her experiences were excluded from discussions with the doctors.

In the second pattern, Marylou Long and Maria Martinez were as unaware as the doctor that contextual information was important. Both women with the help of their doctors made reproductive-related decisions that when examined in a broader, contextual framework may not have been in their best interests.

In the final pattern, both Sally Barrett and Amanda Adams consciously withheld relevant information from their doctors. Unlike Maria Martinez and Corinne Conrad, they trusted their views enough to override medical advice but not enough to challenge their doctors. Instead these women made their own decisions behind their doctors' backs and (1) would be labeled noncompliant by their doctors—an opinion reinforced in medical literature—and (2) did not receive adequate medical care, which they were paying for. Doctors are confident that they know best. Patients' interpretations are not seen as central to the diagnostic-treatment process. In this context Sally Barrett kept her own counsel. She bowed to her doctor's expertise interactionally but made her own decisions. Similarly, Amanda Adams, who was uncomfortable discussing her reproductive concerns with her male doctor, did nothing to inform his ignorance. The doctor not only assumed that she complied with his medical advice but also was left with his ideal of the medical relationship intact.

For the most part, all of these women, whether satisfied or not, compliant or not, were unaware that the information they had was of importance for good health care. Medical understanding and good care were at stake as well as the women's own understanding of their bodies and reproductive lives. Both the women patients and their doctors were behaving as they had learned to—perhaps they were being good doctors and patients in a bad medical model. For to divide social from biological, mind from body, is a conceptual not an individual error. Human beings are not machines and cannot, try as they might, adhere to such a narrow model. Health is not just a matter of bodily processes. As we have seen, social information is crucial to good health.

Although doctors negate the social, contextual information that people try to insert into medical discussions, they unexaminedly accept their own social knowledge—their views of appropriate reproductive behavior and proper roles for women. The difference here is that women's social information is defined as subjective and essentially unnecessary for proper health care, yet doctors' social assumptions are taken for granted or, if considered at all, seen as related to good health care. The three patterns discussed show this clearly. Whether women consciously tried to insert contextual information as was represented in Pattern 1, were unaware that it was relevant to their health as in Pattern 2, or intentionally withheld it as in Pattern 3, their understanding of their lives in relation to their bodies was assumed inappropriate to the medical encounter. Doctors' societal attitudes toward women and toward what is considered scientific prevailed. Medical dominance in a hierarchical system sustained and is sustained by a scientific world view that corresponds to the interests of those in power. On one hand, doctors dominate the field of health care as they prevail interactionally with patients. Their role as experts allows them to do so very consciously. On the other hand, and more subtly, the underlying model has influenced the assumptions of both women and doctors so that both envision health care in very limited terms.

REPRODUCTION AND MEDICAL SCIENCE

At this point the questions might be asked: Why focus on women patients? Hasn't the medical model affected all patients? The rise of scientific medicine certainly has affected health care delivery for both men and women. But sexuality and reproduction place women at special risk. A masculinist science and the cultural authority of scientific medicine define women and treat their bodily processes as diseases in need of medical control. Yet the reproductive activities of women, in their experiences, are not diseases or necessarily physical breakdowns. Reproduction and sexuality cannot be conceptualized as some diseases have been, purely in terms of physiological mechanisms. Rather, they are a part of women's ongoing activities in social and personal life. In an obvious and immediate sense, reproduction and sexuality involve women's bodies and biology, but just as obviously they also involve a woman's sense of self, her relationship with others and with her family, her connections with social mores and with cultural beliefs. The dualism inherent in the modern view of human beings divides women's bodies from their social lives. In part this dualism reflects scientific assumptions that conceptualize and approach physical phenomena in terms of biophysiological mechanisms. If this approach is combined with definitions of and attitudes toward women, the tenacity of the scientific-medical approach to understanding and treating women's bodies is more understandable.

Women were aligned with nature and reproduction in a new, scientific way; in fact, they were reduced to these functions. Once women were defined as primarily reproducers and reproduction was defined as a biological process in need of expert care, the medical institution was in line to take control.

It is here that science, medicine, and reproduction come together. In the scientific world view, women and nature need to be tamed. In the medical model reproduction is managed. Taming and controlling are defined as masculine. The shift to a scientific world view was accompanied by a concomitant shift in medicine from women helpers and midwives to male doctors and surgeons. Although this transition was slow and has been tied to the many social, economic, and political changes in Europe and America, a scientific view complemented these changes and allowed the new medicine to claim scientific supremacy. The ability to intervene and master the whims of nature supported the mastering of disease and childbirth. Indeed, childbirth was defined as a disease in need of management by the new medical experts (see Chapter 2). Doctors offered an interventionary, pain-free childbirth, and women understandably turned to them. This shift started with affluent women and then spread. In the nineteenth century childbirth was often a hardship. The hope that medical intervention could decrease the risk and pain was worth pursuing. But the pursuit was costly. Women sought help in controlling their bodies, but medicine became yet another institution in the social control of women.[6]

Reproduction, production, and sexuality are biological processes, but reproduction has been limited to the material (O'Brien 1981), and production and sexuality have been inundated with social commentary. Marx, after all, derived the bulk of his work from human needs to produce, and Freud's studies on the complexities of eros are the foundation for his life's work. What does this contradiction mean for the definition of biology? Ruth Hubbard, a biologist, addresses this question: "We have no way of knowing what people's 'real' biology is, because the concept has no meaning. . . . People's biology develops in reciprocal and dialectical relationships with the ways in which we live. Therefore human biology cannot be analyzed or understood in social isolation" (1983:6–7).[7]

So for Hubbard biology is inseparable from its social context. Yet modern medicine, a biological science, continues to isolate itself from any cultural or historical understandings. It also is generalized to cover all individuals. A glaring example of medical generalization can be found in the current controversy over cesarean births. Although no one would deny that in some cases a cesarean section is the safest delivery for the health and lives of both mother and baby, many argue that this procedure is widely overused. In 1983, 20.3 percent of all U.S. births were delivered by cesarean section. In Massachusetts, hospitals varied from a 7.63 percent to 31.22 percent cesarean birth rate. "Given the fact that there are places with high-risk mothers and babies that have good outcomes and lower cesarean rates, this does throw the burden of justification on the doctors and institutions with high cesarean rates" (Knox, *Boston Globe*, October 21, 1984). This rate has continued to grow.

Is this increasing cesarean rate a physiological necessity? Many factors, some social, some biological, have been used to explain the steady increase of this procedure.

Dr. Waldo Fielding, an obstetrician-gynecologist and frequent speaker on women's health, advocates cesareans based on a surprising physiological view of women and reproduction: "The female anatomy is not made to have babies. She was designed to be a four-legged animal. Instead she stands on two feet, so the entire weight of pregnancy doesn't hang free, but sits on the large vessels, causing fluid to build up in her extremities. . . . Furthermore, there isn't a cervix owned by any woman that doesn't tear" (Knox and Karagianis, *The Boston Globe*, October 21, 1984). Women, though defined as reproducers, are not made to reproduce. Women's bodies, defined as machines, are defective. On one hand, women have been reduced to their biological functions, and on the other hand, these functions, through the capricious whim of nature, are inadequate and in need of expert intervention, surgeries, and doctors to make them functional.

In addition to physiological explanations, social accounts for the high cesarean rates abound. Doctors say their practice has been influenced by a changing social context. They fear that if anything goes wrong, they will be sued. High rates of malpractice suits encourage early intervention; more money is to be made from a high-tech surgical rather than a low-tech vaginal delivery; scheduled cesareans are more convenient for doctors and hospital staffs than the unpredictable vaginal birth. In addition, the definition of a normal birth is a social construct. In the 1950s scales delineating the appropriate time schedules for the stages of a "normal" delivery became part of hospital routine. In the past decade they have shortened. However defined, these scales are intended to be approximate, but doctors often abide by them carefully. They are seen as the norm—a fact—and the woman whose labor is different becomes deviant, requiring intervention. Thus individual difference between laboring mothers is less likely to be allowed. Childbirth/nature must be made to conform one way or another (Rothman 1982).

Women, seen as dysfunctional, lose rights over and rapport with their own bodies. They become concerned with every change because their bodies have become high-risk, out-of-control objects. Women obsessed in this way need constant checkups, perpetuating their reliance on experts. The diseasing of reproduction not only creates fears in women, it also produces dependence on the medical profession, increasing medical authority. Although this affects all women, regardless of class or status, it also separates them. As patients with individually diseased bodies, women are locked into a medical approach. Isolated in this way, it is more difficult for women to find solidarity based on shared reproductive interests.

If reproduction is a meeting of biological and social historical meanings, how can we understand the continued insistence that it is a biological fact, narrowly defined? It is my contention that to unravel this question we must return to the divisions introduced and later refined by the scientific revolution, which defined technology as a tool to conquer a decontextualized nature. I am not arguing that there exist no differences between nature and society, mind and body, but rather to encourage a cognitive shift to see the intricate, inseparable connections between these dichotomous categories. The world and people are not machines. To continue to see them as such is to perpetuate a mechanical conception of the world as a social fact rather than as a social theory open to reexamination, revision, and criticism.

What does this mean for women and health care? Scientific conceptualizations and medical interventions place the medical profession in a very important position. For it is medicine that primarily legitimizes the current view of reproduction and the emphasis on the biological body/organ. It is medicine that has institutionalized a fairly abstract Cartesian dualism, as it has made the body the domain of conventional health care. Women, defined by their bodies, are particularly at risk in such a narrow model—a risk increased by the diseasing of reproduction.

IDEOLOGY AND FEMINIST SCHOLARSHIP

In recent years feminist scholars have changed the focus from the history of great men and events to the experiences and perceptions of regular women. This is a difficult task because an entrenched ideology about women is often very different from the reality of their everyday experiences."It is important to be aware that the *ideology* of women's nature can differ drastically from, and indeed be antithetical to, the *realities* of women's lives. In fact, the ideology often serves as a smokescreen that obscures the ways women live by making people (including women) look away from the realities or ask misleading questions about them" (Hubbard 1983:3).

The distinction between ideology and realities is particularly relevant to the discussion of women and reproductive care. When women become patients, they become subjects, but the reality of their subjective lives is denied by the ideology of the medical model; the experiential is sacrificed to the bare biological fact. Yet women's biology, while not women's totality, is an ongoing experiential part of daily life. A model that promotes such distinctions mystifies, creating conflict between medical definitions and lived experiences. My conversations with women to expand their doctor interviews highlights this mystification. Corinne Conrad, suspicious that her divorce had affected her health and not helped by the medical approach to amenorrhea, nonetheless accepted the doctor's dismissal of connections between her body and her social life. Maria Martinez was confused about her birth control history and her options but shared the same assumptions that her doctor held. Marylou Long did not think she was confused, but when her life situation was reintegrated into biotechnical information, a shift in perspective became possible. Amanda Adams and Sally Barrett, unable to use their medical care to best advantage, still felt that their doctors and care were excellent. They were able to hold onto the value of their own experiences, but they did so at the risk of medical disapproval—a disapproval neither wanted to confront within a system both were still dependent on. Women, as active agents in their reproduction and health care, and doctors, as dispensers of that care, are playing cards without a full deck.

The effects of the medical model go further than just health care. On the personal level, consciousness is affected. On the societal level, social and political theory is involved. The rise of medical, scientific explanations made it possible to reduce women to their biological parts. Reproduction was once and for all put in its biological place and relegated to medicine. Political theories have concentrated on the human world, not nature. In this view women equaled reproduction, which equaled nature, which in turn did *not* equal a politically relevant group or process worthy of a place in social or political theory. Social thinkers, long interested in the activities of men, were given a rationale for basing this tendency in scientific truth. Medical definitions of women and biology have strengthened this rationale. For if reproduction is solely biological, then it is medicine's domain, not an area for the work of social theorists. Production, not reproduction, men not women, are the focus for studying and understanding social arrangements. The medical model provides yet another verification that women and their roles are unimportant.

This is not to say that women have simply accepted these "truths." On the contrary, several waves of women's movements, the latest still in progress, have challenged societal roles, contributing social theories of their own. Nevertheless, the mystifying effects of abstract, hard-to-grasp cultural assumptions—concretized in social and medical theories and practices—serve to impede progress.

CONCLUSION

Health care is a series of relationships. Starting at its heart, the doctor-patient relationship, we can examine varied dimensions to get a broader picture of this delivery system. In the interaction are demographic variables such as sex, race, class, and age, long considered to have an impact on people's health needs and their health care. For example, Maria Martinez, a poor woman on Medicaid, defined as having enough babies for a state aid case, was offered a contraceptive method that is considered dangerous and was rarely used with other patients in the clinic. It is well documented that different categories of patients receive different care (see Conrad and Kern 1986). Moving out further to the institutional arrangements of medicine, the history of medicine in the United States details the rise of corporate medicine and the development of the medical-industrial complex of drug, insurance, and supply companies, high-tech industries, hospitals, and the AMA. This history suggests that our medical system is based on the dollar as much as on health. Cultural attitudes toward women and reproduction pervade society in general and medicine in particular. Medicine plays a dual role here—it is both influenced by society's definitions of women and doing more than its fair share to maintain those definitions. Finally, moving on to the most abstract cultural layer, that of a scientific world view, the epistemological underpinnings of this world view complement and legitimate many aspects of the doctor-patient relationship. This can be seen for patients whether they are men or women, whether in the office for the treatment of disease or advice on reproduction. It may be arguable that the skier breaking her or his leg needs only a technical fix, but many health and illness issues cannot be separated from contexts that are social, cultural, and political.

When, for example, a friend developed bursitis in his shoulder, he felt his life falling apart. His main passion as well as his livelihood was playing the piano, an activity now difficult because of pain. He complained to and questioned the doctor about this pain. The doctor gave him pain pills to quell what he thought were the major fears—physical discomforts. The medication only mildly reduced the pain, adding the problem of mental haziness. The doctor focused his well-meaning expertise on the shoulder and pain; the patient thought only of what this pain meant for his work and art. The doctor and the patient met for treatment, guided by differing implicit assumptions never made explicit. This chasm was not caused by a conspiracy of secrecy, but it is too wide and too deep to cross easily.

Patients of both sexes are treated within a problematic model. Women, however, as the major recipients of medical treatment for well care, present a unique problem. Not only is reproduction not a disease, try as one may to make it so, it is also a process laden with social, political, and moral connotations for women and society. Given the power of economic and patriarchal assumptions in our society, intertwined as they are with scientific values, doctors' power to control becomes all the more formidable.

NOTES

1. Few professions are allowed such autonomy and self-regulation as doctors and scientists. One of the controversies to emerge in the recent malpractice crises has been the self-regulation of doctors. Many argue that the evidence shows a reluctance on the part of doctors to discipline their own, leading to repeated offenses on the part of incompetents in the profession.

2. Objectivity and the scientific method are questioned here, but the nature of facts is not. Latour and Woolgar (1979) take this argument a step further. They ask us to raise our index of suspicion to the facts themselves. In examining the processes of scientific discovery they argue that facts are constructed in discursive practices as scientists do their work.

3. This paragraph was originally written by Sue Fisher and myself for the introduction to *Gender and Discourse*, ed. Alexandra Dundas Todd and Sue Fisher (Norwood, N.J.: Ablex, 1987). It is included here with the permission of Sue and Ablex. I am indebted to them both.

4. This is a well-worn theme in philosophy—Plato, philosopher-kings, shadows in the cave, and so forth. But the emphasis has changed from the need for a select few who have the ability to rule the state to a select few who can uncover the secrets of the universe through objective, scientific methods.

5. For example, overuse of antibiotics in cattle feed has led to a dangerous strain of bacteria showing up in people who eat the beef. Overuse of antibiotics has been causing health concerns for the elderly, who get stronger infections as bacteria become immune to antibiotics. Furthermore, medicine is an inexact science. McKinlay (1981) argues that medicine is not scientific *enough* and that many discoveries and treatments lack quality-controlled testing. Thus medicine claims to be scientific when it is not and we need it to be, while at the same time relying on and assuming scientific concepts to foster a model not always in patients' best interests.

6. Medical social control has been experienced differently by women of different classes and races as well as individually. My point in dwelling on science here, however, is that it has affected all of medicine at an abstract level, thus all patients, especially women.

7. At some level we have no language even to talk about these connections. By even discussing their connection, we imply separate realms. Thus our very language, reflecting the scientific age, discriminates against women because women are at an even greater disadvantage when mind is separated from body in understanding their own bodies and reproduction.

6 | Across a Crowded Room: Some Problems, Some Solutions

Doctors and patients face each other across a crowded room—a room filled with individual assumptions, organizational contexts, and social, cultural, and political constructs. One aim of this book has been to detail the different aspects of face-to-face encounters between doctors and patients. I have argued that the organization of the profession, the economic structure of society, cultural assumptions about women, and science as a world view can be observed in the examining room between intimate adversaries.

Americans rely on health care relationships that are fraught with conflict. An especially pervasive problem facing both doctors and patients is the lack of systematic understanding that conflicts even exist. After all, this is not the more overt adversarial relationship between law enforcer and lawbreaker, jailer and prisoner, judge and accused. Rather, it is a subtler relationship between healer and the ill, between the dispenser and the seeker of care, in a mutually consensual, if problematic, relationship. Knowledge about these subtle dynamics is crucial if we are to effect change.

Having reviewed in this book problems for the doctor-patient relationship, we are left with the question, Is there any hope? Is there hope that one day the Maria Martinezes can assume that their birth control concerns will be listened to without interruption and be heard in light of their own particularistic experiences? Is there hope that the Marylou Longs will be able to participate in more conscious discussions with doctors and receive enough information to demand more options? Is there hope that the Sally Barretts will not feel compelled to seek medical advice, ignore it, and then deceive their doctors that they are doing so? These are timely questions. Modern medicine is undergoing rapid change.

Howard Waitzkin suggests ways to conceptualize these changes. He discusses change in medicine as inextricably entwined with the structure of the larger society. He argues that "health reforms that do not address the relationships between the health system and the broader social structure are doomed to failure" (1983:5). He goes on to distinguish between "reformist" change, which addresses care but leaves untouched the larger political-economic levels of society, and "nonreformist" change, which attempts to reorganize power structures through political activism. It is here that the analysis of a scientific world view discussed in this book becomes important. Change, whether reformist or nonreformist, requires broad, conceptual understanding of the problems at hand. Analysis of the cultural conditions of science can contribute to this understanding.

My aim in this book has been to make clear the extent of the problems so that patients, medical staff, and policy makers can be better equipped to move in progressive directions. Solutions, ever elusive, will continue to emerge as new angles are analyzed and groups work together. I will conclude with a few examples of how people and organizations are currently coping with these questions, indicating pitfalls to be sidestepped and benefits to be sought. These examples primarily address changes from reformist perspectives; individual and group health may be improved, but the model of medicine and the economic structure of American society go largely untouched. Movement toward nonreformist change is evident in reforms such as the women's health movement, but these changes remain difficult to achieve. Whether striving for reformist or nonreformist change, however, conceptual clarity is vital, for people continue to wrestle with an entrenched health care system.

COALITIONS AND OPPOSITIONS

Depending on who is targeted as the problem, solutions take varying forms. Cozy coalitions have appeared between historically estranged bedfellows, and equally unexpected antipathy has emerged among old friends.

Doctors and Patients

David brought his son Ben to see the pediatrician for vague but persistent health problems—sporadic fevers, headaches, intestinal disturbances. For several years the family had belonged to a health maintenance organization (HMO) offered through David's work. The doctor had provided satisfactory care for all of the three children since the family joined this program. After a thorough examination and discussion of various possibilities with David, the doctor referred Ben to a specialist outside of the HMO for further investigation. To refer a patient to an outside doctor, the pediatrician was required to submit his request to an HMO administrator. David was assured that this was a routine procedure.

Sarah found herself unexpectedly in surgery for an infection in her leg. She belonged to a health care organization affiliated with a hospital in her area. After the first surgery it was found that gangrene had set in and her stay in the hospital was prolonged. After a second surgery, the doctor assigned to Sarah ordered physical therapy to ease her discomfort and help her become ambulatory.

Marian, suffering chronic anxiety attacks, sought the help of a psychiatrist. The doctor explained her options: short-term psychological therapy combined with drug therapy or long-term psychological therapy without drugs. Marian and the doctor decided on the latter.[1]

In the above cases the expected administrative compliance based on medically perceived patients' needs was not forthcoming. All of the doctors were surprised. The HMO, reversing past policy, vetoed outside services in favor of in-house care except in extreme emergencies. Ben's doctor protested that the tests and expertise needed were not available at the HMO. He was told to do the best he could. Sarah's doctor was told that she would probably lose the leg so why bother with a physical therapist. Although the psychiatrist argued against drugs as the therapy of choice, he was overruled, after several therapy sessions, by Marian's insurance company, which argued that she could be equally well served by drugs (cutting costs).

Doctors and hospitals have traditionally gone together like two peas in a pod. The patient has been the problem—complaining, not getting well, not paying bills, not complying with doctors' orders and hospital routines. Increasingly, physicians, like Dr. Arthur Relman of the *New England Journal of Medicine* in television interviews and medical journal editorials, and Dr. Sidney M. Marchasin, in newspaper editorials, criticize the rise of medical commercialism, the new blatancy of profit mongers in the form of "investor-owned health chains," and the effects of these innovations on the doctor-patient relationship.

Historically we have regarded health care as a community enterprise, a social responsibility undertaken for the common good. Now that is changing: Wall Street has discovered that health care is a major growth industry. . . . The investor-owned hospital would be answerable not to community leaders or the local medical profession, but to remote executive officers, financial managers and investors whose main concern is the bottom line of the profit-and-loss statement. . . . But even the authority and independence of the physician is coming under siege. A measure now being studied in the Legislature (Senate bill 2284) would permit hospitals to hire (and, it follows, to fire) doctors. . . . It threatens to compromise the historic tradition of the physician being the patient's advocate, and would invite the commercial exploitation of patients by profit-seeking institutions. (Marchasin, *Los Angeles Times*, August 1, 1984)

At issue here is patient care and physicians' independence. Even though physicians are the last great bastion of professional autonomy and have the strongest union around (the American Medical Association) to protect their interests, they may find themselves turned into wage earners selling their labor in the interests of corporate profits. Medical inflation, out of hand for some time, has come under attack from consumers—the individual patient, government, and employers alike (all of whom have been paying higher and higher insurance premiums and health care costs). This attack has forced some control on a previously unfettered, upward-moving spiral. Enter corporate medicine.

The American Medical Association, which spends most of its protective energy keeping government interference at bay, has unwittingly left the back door open to corporate takeovers. When Humana started an ever-expanding chain of lucrative hospitals, its president wanted the firm "to provide as uniform and reliable a product as a McDonald's hamburger coast to coast" (in Starr 1982:431). McDonald's may not provide much in the promotion of health, but it is certainly a model of standardization, efficiency, and profit.

Physicians are not in danger of becoming "proletarianized" or automatons on the assembly line of surgery, geared solely to the whims of big business, but they may have to start following more of a company plan, with tighter controls than have previously been in place. In the past doctors have been the primary decision makers for health care practices. Accountability, when present, was primarily to peer groups and within their own hospitals and practices. Doctors decided what patients to admit, how to treat them, what procedures were necessary, and how long patients would remain in care. In the words of one hospital manager, "Those days are gone forever." Today insurance companies and regulating agencies demand an accountability unheard-of in the past. Many decisions are now regulated by utilization managers outside and inside the hospital. Doctors' decision-making power, though still an important factor, has been considerably decreased.

For example, in California the medical staff of a hospital has taken its own administration to court in a hospital privilege case. The medical staff found a surgeon unqualified for practice in the hospital. They were concerned that this doctor would jeopardize patient care. The decision was based on medical board complaints against the surgeon for fourteen acts of "gross negligence" and performing unnecessary and excessive surgery.

He was also the defendant in eight current malpractice suits. The administrative board of the hospital overruled the medical staff's decision and added the surgeon to the hospital's roll of doctors. This particular doctor fills beds. He advertises himself as the "bloodless surgeon" specializing in surgery to groups such as Jehovah's Witnesses, who refuse to accept blood transfusions. The dispute is whether hospital doctors or administrators control who is admitted to the hospital staff, traditionally the former's decision. The California Medical Association strongly stated, "Hospitals face great financial pressure. . . . The businessmen who run some hospitals will be under great pressure to put physicians on the staff who can fill empty beds, and there will be pressure to overlook necessary qualifications. This isn't good for patients and it isn't good medicine" (Parachini, *Los Angeles Times*, July 27, 1984).

Doctors, like Marchasin, are publicly decrying big business's growing influence over health care. Genuine concern for patients and quality of care runs throughout these debates. It seems that patients and doctors might be allies after all, but the patient needs to view these power struggles with a skeptical eye. The above quotations raise many issues. Such descriptions as "community enterprise," the "common good," and "patient advocate" applied to doctors' attitudes toward patients ring a little hollow given the historical development of the health care system. The image of a profit-oriented corporate bully blustering into a humanistic, caring arena seems slightly askew. Certainly, a more pronounced emphasis on profit is a hazard for health care, especially for the poor. Although corporate control is reorganizing health care, the role of money and profit is not a new problem in this system. Profit has always been a part of American medicine. The AMA has vigorously defended this aspect of medicine, fighting against government programs and socialized or nationalized health care. There has, in modern medicine, always been a two-class delivery system, with the poor underserved. Corporate power has consistently played a major role, from the extremely lucrative drug companies, hospital supply companies, and high-tech industries to the insurance conglomerates. The new aspect is that hospitals, traditionally nonprofit and bastions of doctors' professional autonomy, are shifting to a profit orientation, run by business school graduates rather than medical men. Doctors' autonomy is threatened, their financial accountability is increased, and though they are not in danger of becoming totally subservient to these organizations, their professional power is at risk.

Increased accountability of medical care is important. Doctors' under-regulated power is a problem in our health care system. This new accountability, however, focuses not on the care or needs of patients or an improved health delivery but on the costs. The Diagnostic Related Groups

(DRGs) being used in Medicare have been designed to increase account-ability and cut costs. They could do just that, but such measures also have the potential to standardize care to the extent that doctors may find themselves unable to consider individual patients' best interests. Costs need to be cut, but at whose expense? Despite isolated accounts when DRGs have helped or hurt patients, doctors, and the medical system, it will be some time before the benefits and risks can be longitudinally assessed.

How will the doctor-patient relationship fit into these changes? Will people become, even more than they are already, a collection of parts to be quickly and profitably shuttled down the assembly line? Will they be the ones to be proletarianized in the interests of cutting costs? Will the doctor-patient relationship, already in trouble, become increasingly a fast-health service, ever more impersonal even if doctors want to be caring providers?

Jeff Goldsmith, an economist, offers a more optimistic view of the important role the public will play in these changes. He suggests that based on the impending oversupply of doctors[2] and economic changes, doctors' power is at risk in yet another way. He argues, "The patient will no longer be what one famous health services analyst called the 'breathing brick' of the health care system. Consumer sovereignty will be a watchword of the competitive health care system" (1981:24). Goldsmith argues that in the past doctors practiced in a seller's market. Feedback from patients did not have to be taken too seriously. Today, however, the seller's market is dwindling, and a consumer's market is rising. Goldsmith asserts that doctors will increasingly find themselves in the new position of having to take patients' needs seriously.[3]

Examination of the rise in malpractice suits points further to the need for the medical profession to pay closer attention to patients' concerns. Malpractice suits have been on the rise with huge sums of money awarded annually for physical and mental grief. In consequence, medical insurance premiums have risen dramatically. These enormous premiums and malpractice awards are felt by both practitioners and the public.

Doctors are justified in fighting such sharp rises in malpractice costs in and out of the courtroom; but medical mistakes happen frequently (see Bosk 1979). The public needs protection, too. Derek Bok's report on medical education and clinical medicine cites a study that found a 22 percent diagnostic error rate in a survey of one hundred autopsies at a leading teaching hospital. "In almost half of these instances, a correct diagnosis would have indicated a change in the treatment that might have prolonged life" (1984:6). Self-policing and professional loyalty by doctors too often allow incompetence and negligence to go unchecked, hurting both competent doctors and patients.

Incompetence and negligence aside, the interesting question is why some people sue their doctors following medical mismanagement but others do not. What leads some to the courts and not others? Doctors and lawyers loudly debate the role the ever-expanding legal profession has played in encouraging malpractice escalation. The public is criticized for greed and expectations of perfection. But another factor points to the importance of communication between doctors and patients.

"To err is human" is a statement rarely applied to medical mistakes, but it appears likely to be said by patients who have been satisfied with how their doctors treated them. In other words, when Peggy Cass's doctor operated on the wrong knee and then said something to the effect of "Oh well, it needed surgery anyway," Cass went straight to the New York courts (*Boston Globe*, September 22, 1985). Evidence shows that patients are less likely to take this route when doctors show concern rather than indifference about their medical errors.

Medical mistakes can range from the merely inconvenient to the difference between life and death. Many of the malpractice cases for these mistakes seem justified (for example, the wrong knee was operated on). The resultant loss of health or life requires compensation. But many suits as well as the mistakes themselves could be avoided with adequate communication. The courts become a place (often the only place) for people to retaliate against the power and indifference they feel from the medical profession. It is an expensive solution. The costs are most immediately felt by doctors. In the long run, however, they find their way back to patients in the form of increased insurance premiums, higher deductibles, and decreased services. An improved doctor-patient relationship in which patient felt respect and care in the medical system could provide, first, a decrease in medical mistakes and, second, an alternative, in some cases, to the law courts. It may seem out of place to raise malpractice issues in a discussion of possible alliances between doctors and patients, but an alliance here would decrease some of the reasons for present animosity.

Power blocs in the medical system are facing a reorganization of allies. The traditionally aligned professional groups can find themselves looking at each other from opposite sides of the table. To lament the loss of health care as a community enterprise may be misstating the case. It is important, however, to note that whether the reason be a true interest in the patient or a fear of loss of power or rise in malpractice, doctors may increasingly see the patient as a potential partner in this new struggle.

For segments of the medical industry—AMA, hospitals, corporations—this struggle is one of power, money, and control. For patients it is more immediate; at times it will be a question of life and death, and for all it will be a question of health. American medical consumers need to be aware, more acutely than before, of the role they can play, the demands they can make, before choosing who and where to align themselves in the present reshuffling. As the research literature shows, people have reported many dissatisfactions with their medical care. Perhaps the time is ripe to voice these dissatisfactions more systematically. Perhaps the time has come when doctors will find it in their interests to listen more reflectively to patients and the public both inside and outside of the office, clinic, or hospital.

> *Benefits:* What has been a subtly conflictual relationship between doctors and patients could move toward a closer alliance. Patient groups could gain power as sought-after consumers.

> *Risks:* Business administrators, with an eye always on the dollar, could curtail quality of health care, frustrating doctors and adversely affecting patients. In sum, the coalition of doctors and patients would not be strong enough to fight corporate America effectively. Or the medical profession and hospital chains could settle their differences, forming an even stronger coalition against increased patient demands.

Big Business and Health Care Plans

Since the 1930s, and especially since World War II, American industry has offered employees comprehensive health care coverage. Starting as a "fringe" benefit making up a small percentage of employees' income, it has become a major expense for employers. Big business, which traditionally accepted costs as outlined by the health industry, has begun to protest cost increases. Negotiations over health care have become a major issue between employers and employees, with the former making it clear to the health sector that the costs must come down. Lee A. Iacocca, Chrysler Corporation chair, has warned that the high costs of health care coverage for Chrysler workers are threatening America's ability to compete with foreign manufacturers. General Motors claims that the cost of health insurance for employees adds $430 to the price of each new car. General Motors's health insurance rates have increased 15 percent per year for the last ten years, and abuses by medical professionals are thought to be common (Risen, *Los Angeles Times*, August 16, 1984).

The insurance companies, pressured by industry, have passed the squeeze on to medicine. Organized medicine in Massachusetts, in a suit against Blue Shield, lost the right of balance billing, to bill Blue Shield subscribers beyond the insurer's payment. Furthermore, the governor of the state introduced legislation and won a ban on balance billing. The Massachusetts Medical Society claims that a free market in services will ensure the best quality care and lower prices, but the courts, insurance company, and state government do not agree (Knox, *Boston Globe*, November 29, 1984).

The demands of industry for medical care could open new possibilities for patient care or present new risks. With employers demanding more accountability, patients could gain clearer understanding of what is really needed and what is not. A reduction in unnecessary surgeries, tests, and so forth could cut both costs to the consumer and iatrogenic (doctor-induced) illness. Concomitantly, the worker must be aware that such stringent cutbacks could also decrease quality of health care.

A few glimmers of hope in this area have appeared. General Motors and the United Auto Workers in their recent contract bargaining seem to have made some headway toward more cost-effective but comprehensive health coverage. Workers are to be allowed to choose between several programs including an HMO, a network of designated health care professionals, and a traditional insurance plan with General Motors continuing to cover the entire cost.

Consultant firms have organized to help facilitate health care packages for industry focusing on decreasing medical cost and increasing medical accountability for costs and care. One such firm, Affordable Health Concepts, in Sacramento, California, has worked extensively with labor union and industry negotiations. Its approach combines, in the firm's words, traditionally conservative and radical tactics to produce reasonably priced, adequate coverage. From a conservative perspective it has hospitals bid on health care contracts. Competition is encouraged to drive the costs down. From a more radical perspective doctors and hospitals are required to provide heightened public reports under the awarded contracts. Conservative and radical policies coincide: financial discipline is imposed, and medical accountability is increased to the *consumer*. More information is delivered, giving people more control over medical decisions. One of the major aims of this firm is to trim the fat of medical care without sacrificing the quality of that care by bringing the recipients of health care into the bargaining room and encouraging more public control. Its emphasis is on short-term goals and tactics. In the long run it is aware that these strategies may not hold as many benefits for the consumer. The claim, however, is that the parameters of health care are changing so fast that long-term strategies become impractical and short-term strategies in today's conditions can provide a strong plus for the public.

In the former section, I discussed the possibility of an alliance between doctors and patients against encroaching corporate power. In this section, the alignment is quite different. The problem is in the medical profession—its lack of accountability to the public and the power enjoyed by hospitals and doctors. This highlights another set of solutions; the players again change sides. Instead of doctors and patients aligning against big business, we see big business and labor unions (potential patients) fighting the medical profession/industry. Once again, it is time to examine all of the options, especially for the public, which has much to gain or much to lose in these strategies.

> *Benefits:* Increased medical accountability is demanded for the public with more stringent medical financial discipline and stronger consumer control for better health care becoming possibilities.

> *Risks:* Employers and health care deliverers could realign to provide cheaper but less adequate and comprehensive health care to employees. The cuts could come in quality of care rather than industry profits.

Both of the coalitions mentioned above offer reformist change. The model of scientific medicine goes unquestioned, and the economic structure of a profit-oriented, unequal health care system is left intact. For the most part these struggles for alliance are struggles among interest groups all fighting for their piece of the pie. The interest groups are the medical profession, big business, hospitals, and consumer groups. Others lack the power to engage in this struggle—unorganized labor, the unemployed, and the working poor continue to be ignored.

MODELS OF MEDICINE

Coalitions among interest groups reflect possible changes in the current health care system that are important for the doctor-patient relationship. At issue is quality of care, which in our system is tied to economics. The research for this book, however, reveals problems that go deeper than economics. Quality of care is tied just as closely to the model of medicine that is built into the very fabric of the American health care system. Changes in this model have been discussed, albeit rarely, yet a problem always remains: what to keep and what to change.

Harold Bursztajn, Richard Feinbloom, Robert Hamm, and Archie Brodsky, a team of doctors, psychologist, and medical writer, have written a book, *Medical Choices, Medical Chances*, outlining some of the problems and possibilities inherent in the model of modern medicine. They label the current model, based on Newtonian science, the mechanistic model. This approach assumes the mind-body dualism, the single cause of disease, reliance on overly technical solutions, and an obsession with certainty. Uncertainty in this model is to be banished at all costs, and sometimes the costs are very high. The authors outline an alternative approach—the probabilistic model—based on the changes brought about in the conceptual shifts introduced in physics by Einstein. This model allows for broader connections among biology, mind, and environment. Disease and health are tied to multicausalities rooted in more complex contexts than the single germ cause. Observation and patience are reintroduced into medical care, decreasing the use of medical technology to cases in which it is really needed. And last, doctors and patients need to learn to cope with uncertainty as a part of science, medicine, and everyday life. They argue that whereas uncertainty has become a routine part of modern physics, modern medicine has been left behind. The medical profession has clung so tenaciously to the scientific, mechanistic model that it becomes vulnerable to the claim that in modern definitions it is being *unscientific*.

We are a society that seeks certainty. We are uncomfortable with the unknown; we want control over our lives. This discomfort is reflected in medicine, with both doctors and patients demanding an answer:

> Just as a patient may seek to evade the unknown future consequences of an illness by simply failing to acknowledge them, so a doctor may do anything to avoid being exposed as uncertain or in error. . . . A woman who fails to perform regular breast self-examinations and a doctor who relies on laboratory readings in place of clinical judgment may both be fleeing from the responsibility of making choices in an uncertain world. . . . One way to avoid the anxiety that accompanies uncertainty is to bury one's head in the sand. Another way is to seek assurance from technology. (Bursztajn et al. 1981:xv)

Both solutions—avoidance and overtreatment—are potentially damaging to our health. These tendencies have deeply entrenched cultural roots that spread to the model of health care and are reflected in the doctor-patient relationship. Bursztajn et al. argue that the fact of uncertainty in life and medicine needs to be faced by doctors and the public if health care is to improve.

In a moving personal story, one of the authors—an intern in a large teaching hospital—tells of K, "a case of uncertainty." A small child, K came to the hospital suffering from malnutrition and was underdeveloped physically and emotionally, with chronic ear infections and immune deficiency. He was treated in two different models of health care. The hospital house staff went into action with tests and medical intervention. Dr. S, the intern, undertook to try different methods—less emphasis on immediate diagnosis, more time gaining the child's confidence and dealing with his eating problems. Investigation into the child's life at home and the context of his illness offered Dr. S further evidence to treat K in as noninterventionary a manner as possible. Dr. S was willing to live with uncertainty until K was strong enough to withstand technological intervention when needed. When under Dr. S's care, K thrived. When left to the hospital's standard procedures, K's health declined, he became more withdrawn, refused to eat, and eventually died.

This example was not used to discredit all use of technology, testing, and modern medical technique. Dr. S wanted technology to work for him and the patient rather than their working for technology. The hospital staff could not stand the uncertainty of not having a diagnosis and a single underlying cause of K's problems (which were not understood even after all the testing). Dr. S, on the other hand, wanted to broaden his understanding of the child's illness by incorporating contextual influences and clinical observation and accepting the complexities and uncertainties inherent in the problem.

Dr. S's story highlights the difficulties of introducing new methods into hospitals and gaining the cooperation of the staff. Throughout the book Dr. S's experiences are used to highlight how to work on this problem—in what circumstances to use the hospital and to avoid it, what doctors and hospitals need to think about to reassess health care, and what patients need to do to encourage constructive changes. Drossman (1983), reporting his clinical work with patients coming to him with gastrointestinal problems, reinforces this view that doctors unrealistically demand certainty in their search for *the* diagnosis. He has found, like Dr. S, that recognition of psychosocial dimensions incorporated into biophysiological investigation leads to improved diagnosis and care, as well as a better doctor-patient relationship.[4]

Other examples of current shifts in medical thinking are slowly gaining acceptance in practice if not by established medicine. Gordon (1984) reports that between 1978 and 1983 the number of holistic health centers in the United States grew from approximately fifty to several hundred. I suspect a more general listing of alternative health providers would show a vastly greater number today.

New approaches have come from mavericks trained as M.D.'s such as clinical ecologists, orthomolecular practitioners, and those interested in behavioral medicine. Alternatives have also come from healers outside conventional medical training such as acupuncturists, chiropractors, nutritionists, Alexander teachers, and so forth. Each of these groups from very different perspectives and using diverse techniques tries to broaden the medical model to include stress factors and in some cases environmental influences. The aim is to promote health (through preventive strategies), not just treat disease. Their increasing popularity could reflect the public's response to medical mistakes, impotence, or both. Certainly most alternative healers deliver a less invasive, more prevention-oriented health care that attracts many. Taylor argues, however, that these are not the only reasons for the growth of the alternative health movement. She finds evidence that an important influence is how people are treated by their doctors. The doctor-patient relationship becomes a key for understanding this flight. "The one consistent theme (in addition to therapeutic failure) in consumers' responses and in observers' speculations is dissatisfaction with the *relationship* which obtains with conventional physicians . . . and the attraction of a different kind of relationship with alternative practitioners" (Taylor 1984:204). Cobb, as early as 1954, found that when cancer patients left their doctors, turning to alternative sources of help, it was because they felt emotionally abandoned by their physicians. They sought the caring provided by alternative healers.

Alternative methods of treatment are extremely varied, but the holistic health movement is committed to a personal orientation lacking in the disease/organ focus of conventional medicine. Whether or not patients are made healthier seems to slide into the background; what comes sharply into focus is patients' demands for respect and concern in the treatment of their unique problems.

> *Benefits:* The medical model and scientific world view present perhaps the most elusive and abstract problems to grasp in health care. These approaches offer beginnings in how to reshape clinical care of patients practically and re-think the medical model. What is offered is a more personal, patient-oriented approach.

> *Risks:* Although raising nonreformist criticisms of a neglected area of our health care system—the model itself—new clinical approaches tend to concentrate on the individual patient rather than political change. In some of the clinical work there is the risk of blaming victims for their health problems—personal lifestyle can be emphasized as the key element of ill health.

MEDICAL EDUCATION

One of the obvious starting points for change within medicine is medical school education. As discussed in Chapter 1, the majority of medical schools reinforce attitudes and practices that gear students toward the conventional models of medicine. A few notable changes in today's medical education, however, raise some optimism.

For example, the Medical College of Wisconsin in Milwaukee offers a preventive medicine class. In this course, each student is assigned a family (volunteers from the county hospital clinics) for whom he or she is responsible throughout the course. This responsibility includes making home visits, understanding contextual issues, and providing primary care and referral services for all members of the household. Clinical experience—

increasingly emphasized in the early years of medical school—starts the first semester, and patient care is considered a central part of the program.

Loyola Medical School in Illinois requires students to participate in a four-year medical ethics and philosophy program along with the general curriculum. Many schools offer medical ethics, but Loyola requires it and offers more depth over time than the usual one-semester, optional course.

Harvard University in 1985 introduced a "New Pathways" curriculum for a small group of first-year medical students. The format focused on problem solving with a close integration of basic and clinical training. Teaching took place in small groups with much self-directed study, individually organized. The program combined this new approach with traditional medical skills in the hope of preparing doctors for future changes in medicine. It has proved so successful that Harvard has now incorporated these changes throughout the medical school curriculum.

Women, 10 percent of medical students in 1970 and 30 percent in 1980, are becoming doctors in growing numbers. Controversy continues to flare over how much their added presence will address problems in the medical system, but it is undeniably a progressive move for women and for societal equity. Minorities, men and women, have not fared so well. People of color, depending on race, make up a minuscule percentage of medical students. Since the *Bakke* decision, schools can choose to admit no minority candidates. This choice is reflected in the decrease in minority medical students in the last decade. Some schools have taken a different strategy. Minority status, open to any race, requires a *demonstrated* commitment to helping those medically underserved because of poverty, geographic location, or both. Thus students who enter under this status bring a more sensitive, primary interest in delivering care to those who need it the most.

To require doctors to be committed to improving health for all is important, but to label this commitment "minority status" is confusing. Minority students continue to be vastly underrepresented. They stand a better chance for acceptance under minority status. Thus when they do reach the medical ranks, they have to be committed and qualified, whereas white students can merely be qualified. Inequality persists. Furthermore, if principles are important, one should not have to achieve minority status to be required to show such qualifications. All incoming students should show *demonstrated* commitment humanistically and technically.

This inequality among those eligible to be trained as doctors also prevails between medical students and the people they learn on. Medical students in training traditionally have their first contact with sick people in public or veterans' hospitals, where the patients are very different from the students. In Wisconsin students learn medical care in a broader environment, but as is usually the case, the patients form an experimental group and most of them are poor. On one hand, it is arguable that these patients need care the most and in this setting they at least get some attention. On the other hand, students learn on the group that is least healthy and least like themselves, which makes it easier to define patients as "other," "different," "inferior," "difficult," and so forth.

> *Benefits:* Some medical schools are slowly expanding their curriculums to include broader questions pertinent to health. Students with a primary commitment to patient care and inequalities in the delivery system are gaining admittance to medical training, heralding some emphasis on progressive change.
> *Risks:* The changes are slow and remain reformist by not challenging the structure of the medical system. Racism, sexism, and elitism still abound, with many schools and faculty holding tenaciously to conventional medical approaches.

DOCTOR-PATIENT COMMUNICATION

Increasingly medical education includes courses in the interviewing and communication skills that doctors will need in medical practice. Video cameras have been placed in examination rooms to provide doctors and residents with tapes of their interactions. Critical viewing of the tapes with colleagues can encourage improved interpersonal skills. Research funding is presently in abundance to investigate the importance of communication skills and how doctors can interact with patients to the best advantage. As the literature discussed in earlier chapters suggests, this is an area in need of such investigation, especially when the patient is a woman.

It has been argued that women often make inadequate patients. It can also be argued that doctors are often incompetent in interpersonal situations. It is true that people need to adjust their behavior in doctors' offices but not necessarily in the ways doctors suggest. It may be true that people, particularly women, need to be less submissive in medical interactions, asking questions that ensure their understanding and their informed agreement in medical decision making, but they also need to challenge structural constraints and learned submission and to gain respect for their own interpersonal skills. They need to learn to push for their right to tell their stories. Doctors need to reassess their long-held, often unexamined attitudes toward women and patients, learning a new language to discuss health issues.

Lazarre and colleagues (1975) found in their work with psychiatric outpatients of both sexes examples of just how needed these changes are. Their research revealed that the doctors dominated the interaction to the extent that patients' requests were often never mentioned. They advocate eliciting the patients' interpretations and requests from the onset of the interview, gearing the interaction toward a negotiation between two active participants rather than the traditional active doctor/passive patient scenario. If the patients can shape the initial direction of the interaction they are more likely to continue to raise topics they consider important. The problem lies in changing the consciousness of both patients and doctors so the former will understand better what topics to raise and the latter will learn a new way of listening.

Interest in adept medical communication is now higher than ever. As the doctor role is redefined to increase interactional competence, it is crucial that public awareness of new possibilities for the patient role also receives adequate attention. Patients, traditionally in the passive role in the medical setting, need to be redefined as active participants. Asking the right questions can radically change medical outcomes. When surgery is advised, the simple question, "Do I have any other options?" can have startling results (Chapter 2).

It is important, when possible, for people to know their options and share information before discussing final decisions with their doctors. Bookstores are filled with self-help literature on how to manage your health inside and outside the doctor's office. A bureau has been organized that for a fee will research information on any specific ailment and send the results.[5] Armed with such knowledge, patients are less likely to be passive. Once again, however, such tactics usually cost money and are thus more available to some groups in society than others.

As doctors receive expanded training in communication skills and patients become more aware of the need for their active participation, perhaps, for some, the struggles described in Chapters 1, 2, and 3 will decrease. The problems discussed in Chapter 4 and elaborated on in Chapter 5, however, require deeper analysis of the changes needed in the doctor-patient relationship. If communication skills alone increase without adequate attention paid to deeper problems in the scientific, medical model, participants, even though becoming more interactionally competent, will do little to improve health care. In fact, the risk exists that if communication alone improves, patients' trust will increase—creating a situation that could be unhealthy.

Daily life, interactions, and communication do not exist in a vacuum. They both influence and are influenced by larger cultural values and societal expectations. Abstract models of medicine and science do not constitute a separate realm disconnected from doctor-patient communication. The form and content of talk is closely tied to larger issues. Thus the problems in the mechanistic model of medicine and in the economic system, *in conjunction* with doctor-patient communication, need reformulation to move toward nonreformist change. All too often each is addressed separately. A wide-angle lens brings into sharp focus the connections between the most micro level of interpersonal communication and the more expansive macro level of cultural assumptions and world views. Bursztajn and his colleagues portray in life-and-death terms the importance of change. Although the consequences presented from my study do not involve such extremes, they do address issues vital to women's lives. Both are deeply tied to quality of life and essential choices for women, men, and children.

> *Benefits:* Increased awareness of the importance of doctor-patient communication presents possibilities for more sensitive doctors and better-informed patients resulting in improved health care. With the chance that doctors' and patients' interests may increasingly coincide, patients' needs and demands are more likely to be met.

> *Risks:* If doctors improve communication skills without broadening their perspective on medicine, patients run a new risk. They may be encouraged further to trust a system that does not always deliver what they need. The earlier statistics on who is helped and who is harmed and who cannot be helped but can be harmed indicate the wide margin for error. If patients are not aware of the depth of the problems, improved medical communication competence alone may enhance their trust, but will this trust be justified?

THE WOMEN'S HEALTH MOVEMENT

The women's health movement has, over the past fifteen years, been a primary influence in the health of women in many countries around the world. The American movement, superbly chronicled by Sheryl Rusek (1978), and international organizations such as ISIS in Switzerland, have had a far-reaching impact on health care delivery to women and women's understandings of their bodies and reproductive lives.

Grass-roots movements, self-help, and strivings for structural change have been important foci for women's health advocates. The first women's self-help clinic opened in Los Angeles in the early 1970s amid legal prosecution and community skepticism. It survived. Similar women's clinics have flourished around the country despite continued harassment from groups on the political right and often the mainstream medical community. For example, the Feminist Women's Health Center in Tallahassee, Florida, suing the Florida Medical Association for monopolizing control of abortions, lost the case but won the battle when on appeal the medical association settled out of court.

In England well woman clinics are slowly being started within the

National Health Service. These clinics focus on the well woman, rather than the ill patient, and are staffed exclusively by women. Katy Gardner (1981), a physician and director of one of the clinics, sees them as a way to promote self-help and move away from the social control of medicalization of women's bodies. Similarly, community clinics such as one in South Boston offer forums entitled "Let's Talk Women to Women," addressing midwifery and routine health care from a self-help, preventive perspective.

The emphasis is on gaining information and control over one's body and health and decreasing reliance on experts. Pauline Bart describes a 1960s illegal abortion center ("Jane") run by feminists in Chicago. She emphasizes the women's abilities to manage all of the work, including performing safe abortions without the assistance of doctors. "For me, the most moving experience was learning how participating in 'Jane' improved the women's self-image and their view of other women, as well as giving them skills which enable them to have more control over their lives" (1981 : 126).

The Boston Women's Health Book Collective has been a major factor in the development of this movement. The continuing success of its self-help book *Our Bodies, Ourselves*, in succeeding editions, bears witness to women's interest in understanding and controlling their health care and lives. The latest edition includes "voices" heard less frequently—women with physical disabilities, aging women, gay women, fat women, and prostitutes. This book is presently in its fourth commercially published American edition with sales in 1984 reaching 2.25 million in English and twelve foreign translations and two more planned (Matchan, *Boston Globe*, September 26, 1984).

Running throughout this book is an emphasis on variety and similarity. All women are different with distinguishable problems. Women of special groups face special obstacles, but all women share certain needs stemming from their position in the society as women and based on bodies that have all too often been controlled by the male medical profession. Esther Rome, one of the book's editors, in an interview to discuss the new edition, stated, "We want women to question what is happening to them." It is argued that the doctor–female patient relationship is characterized by "a profound inequality on every level, an exaggeration of the power imbalance inherent in almost all male-female relationships in our society" (in Matchan 1984 : 62). She even worries that the increasing numbers of female physicians "have absorbed the attitudes of medicine" to be able to practice within the system.

The emphasis of this collective as well as the general flavor of the more than three hundred women's health care groups around the country has been to inform women of their rights and to reeducate them about their bodies. "The bottom line is to move people to take action, to encourage women to not let professional interest groups make decisions about their health and well-being" (Norsigian in Matchan 1984:62).

The women's health movement has advocated reform within and outside of conventional medicine. For example, within the system, the National Women's Health Network with other women's groups has lobbied Congress for health reform in such areas as hazardous contraceptive methods, sterilization abuse, unnecessary surgery, and menopausal treatments using synthetic estrogens. Others have worked with the medical community and sympathetic doctors to improve quality of care for women. Birthing assistants have become common mediators helping women and couples cope with hospital routines and childbirth, keeping hospital intervention to a minimum. Some hospitals have modified their birthing procedures better to suit natural childbirth in response to public demand.[6]

The movement has also advocated change outside of conventional medicine. Self-help and well woman care have grown, often in opposition to accepted medical format. Despite many obstacles, the home birth movement has steadily gained acceptance in parts of the country. Another example of a self-help movement is the Independent Living Movement, started in Berkeley and Boston in the early 1970s by and for the disabled and/or chronically ill. Today there are centers around the country providing consumer resources to turn chronic "patients" into active participants, often outside of conventional medicine. One such center in Boston offers advocacy, education, counseling, training in peer counseling, resources to the disabled community, and consultation on issues of disability to the larger community. Publications such as the *Disability and Chronic Disease Newsletter*, edited by Irving Zola, provide information and sources for research that serve to further collective action and individual control. Alternative medical approaches have found a steady clientele in the chronically ill (men and women) and in women, the two groups most vocally dissatisfied with modern medicine.

The criticisms arising from the women's health movement center on patriarchal power and medical monopoly that dominate not only the theory and practice of medicine but our consciousness as well. The problems women face in medical encounters, whether imposed by insensitive doctors, the organization of modern scientific medicine, or the structure of our society, have been the focus of a change-oriented women's health movement. Scholars and political activists have sought to restructure society, medicine as well as women's roles, with both reformist and nonreformist emphases. Efforts have been made to improve the medical care women receive within the system and to offer alternatives as well as scholarly analyses that work toward structural change. One of this movement's greatest strengths is that mediation has been provided, through books, women's health collectives, and legislation to educate both women and doctors, to facilitate health care choices as a group effort between otherwise isolated individuals, to create coalitions to continue the struggle for change, and always to remember the nature of the battle being fought.

CONCLUSION

Criticisms have ranged from the consideration of doctors examining patients to the wider parameters of the structure of the larger social order. Reforms have had and are having an impact on the health of individuals and some groups in American society. From the growth in community clinics and primary care programs to self-help movements such as women's and workers' health and safety groups to new coalitions, gains have been made. Deeper reforms in the system itself, however, remain elusive. Waitzkin's call for a national health service and the right of all people to have access to health care have been hotly debated but today go largely ignored in policy decisions and in government at the federal level. Questions of what that health care should entail are rarely even debated.[7] In fact, critiques of cultural assumptions and scientific world views in society and medicine are often not even perceived at the level of policy. The emphasis on improving medical care and delivery services within the existing narrow medical model persists as the most accessible avenue to reform. The system—a scientific world view tied to economic interests and conventional attitudes toward women—is left intact. In other words, solutions treat one part of this system just as one organ is the focus of medical care. The carving up of an institution, like the carving up of the body, often seems the most expedient way to treat an acute problem: it appears to offer immediate relief. Unfortunately, this focus leaves the chronic malaise unaddressed and, therefore, unhealed. Changing the *medical model of illness* into a *social model for health*, available to all, raises larger questions all too often ignored or avoided. We hear more about individual responsibility than we do about the need for social change.

Repeatedly, evidence ties health or lack of it more closely to social class, occupation, housing, nutrition, and environment than to available medical services. This does not mean that medical care is not needed. It means that isolated, acute medical care as presently conceived is deeply inadequate. Scientific medicine and society continue to concentrate on illness after the fact, remaining closed to changes in social conditions that create or influence illnesses (see Sidel and Sidel 1984, Waitzkin 1983, and Wright 1982). Nonreformist reforms—changes at the structural level of society—are elusive: "As we strive for short-term reforms and more fundamental long-term change in medicine, we must also strive for basic change in our society, for the movement of our nation and of others toward a world in which we can be just, secure, peaceful, communal, and healthy" (Sidel and Sidel 1984:284).

The development of what is labeled the current crisis in health care, discussed in medical journals, newspapers, government agencies, and academic research, has raised many questions pertinent to all segments of the medical system. Who will control health care? Who will have access to adequate care and who will not? How will these changes affect the doctor-patient relationship? Progressive change, whether of a reformist nature concentrating on one part of the problem or of a comprehensive, nonreformist approach that looks at all of the facets in the larger system, requires increased awareness and collective action to address these questions.

Social movements and coalitions between interest groups offer tentative enlightenment for the delivery of medicine. The stakes are high, and there is much to be gained or lost. The general public particularly needs to know the rules of a new game in which it promises to play a prominent role. Waitzkin, discussing the future of health care in America, concludes, "The present holds little room for complaisance or misguided optimism. Our future health-care system, as well as the social order of which it will be a part, depends largely on the praxis we choose now. . . . Research and analysis must be linked to political action" (1983:238, 214). The choices we make present real dilemmas, for if solutions exist at all, they will not come easily. With each change a new set of problems arises. Involvement in the current system is a must for everyone if we are ever to achieve healthy health care.

My intention in this book has been to raise the issues, to continue the discussion, and thereby to increase knowledge and political activism around health care. Changes are at hand. As discussed on page 1, there is growing skepticism in America about science in general and medicine in particular. Most of these dissatisfactions, however, are expressed as individual complaints. We collectively need a better grasp of the underlying assumptions of our institutions and society, and we need to engage in long-term struggle for public participation in decisions that affect us all. Nothing could be more important—for these are matters of health and sickness, life and death.

NOTES

1. All of these cases are true stories selected from many such experiences reported to me by both patients and doctors.

2. Some argue that the doctor glut is overemphasized. If doctors were redistributed geographically or by specialty (for example, geared toward care of the elderly), perhaps instituting shorter working hours, the glut could be avoided. In other words, we do not have too many doctors, just too many surgeons in places such as San Francisco. In America, however, where practitioners have fought so hard for the freedom to practice unfettered by government influence, changes that seek to relocate doctors geographically—for example, from Boston to a small, rural town or Indian reservation—seem farfetched.

3. The AMA has traditionally kept a tight limit on the numbers of physicians educated in the United States, believing too few were better than too many, if a powerful monopoly is the goal. With the societal and government interest in poverty and the passage of Medicare and Medicaid in 1965, however, medical care, at least theoretically, was to be provided for all those previously denied it. These changes, fiercely fought by the AMA, promised growth in the number of patients. The increasing expenditure of public funds for health care and the expected patient boom, when combined with the limited numbers of physicians, created a problem. Where would the practitioners come from? One solution was to increase the supply of nonphysician providers such as nurses, nurse-practitioners, and physicians' assistants, but the AMA's major forecast called for more doctors. Large amounts of money through the federal Health Manpower Act were spent in anticipation of a doctor shortage. In 1965 there were 88 medical schools with 7,409 graduates in the United States. In 1980 there were 126 medical schools with 15,135 graduates. The number of doctors practicing in 1975 totaled 377,000, growing to 450,000 in 1980, with an estimated 600,000 expected by 1990. This growth has been accompanied by an increase in foreign-trained doctors and a concomitant slowdown in general population growth, with essentially stabilized use of medical services in 1971. The doctor surplus could be as high as 185,000 by 1990. In a 1979 survey 57 percent of doctors practiced in offices that worked at full capacity. Of the remaining 43 percent, one-fourth wanted more work than they had (in Starr 1982). It appears that the power doctors have held onto for so long based on intentionally maintained low numbers of graduates is in jeopardy.

4. Drossman reports that patients often resist this psychosocial incorporation, with questions such as "Is it all in my head?" Since his patients have chronic, often unexplainable health problems, this concern could indicate that they previously had been told their problems were psychogenic. Whatever the reason for such fears, patients' reluctance shows how the public has internalized the idea that illness is located in either the mind or the body. Such strong distinctions that run throughout our society make change all the more difficult.

5. This organization is Planetree Health Resource Center, 2040 Webster Street, San Francisco, California, 94115.

6. Birthing centers in hospitals are tremendously varied. Some provide extensive and progressive care; others provide little more than a name in ordinary hospital settings to reassure the public. Many women's health advocates have argued that the reason hospitals have opened birthing rooms is to recapture a restless population and maintain control of birth in a fight against midwifery and reproductive options.

7. Nationalized or socialized medicine, or universal health insurance (Massachusetts), do broaden access to the present model of care and can offer great benefits to those now denied them. If the model of medicine goes unquestioned, however, the result could be an even more consolidated and problematic approach to health.

Bibliography

Arditti, R., R. D. Klein, and S. Minden, eds. 1984. *Test-Tube Women: What Future for Motherhood?* London: Pandora Press.

Armitage, K. J., et al. 1979. "Responses of Physicians to Medical Complaints in Men and Women." *Journal of the American Medical Association* 241 (May 18):2186–87.

Arms, S. 1975. *Immaculate Deception.* Boston: Houghton Mifflin.

Austin, J. L. 1962. *How to Do Things With Words.* Cambridge, Mass.: Harvard University Press.

Barker-Benfield, G. J. 1976. *The Horrors of the Half-Known Life.* New York: Harper & Row.

Barrett, M., and H. Roberts. 1978. "Doctors and Their Patients: The Social Control of Women in General Practice." In C. Smart and B. Smart, eds., *Women, Sexuality and Social Control.* London: Routledge & Kegan Paul.

Bart, P. 1981. "Seizing the Means of Reproduction: An Illegal Feminist Abortion Collective—How and Why It Worked." In H. Roberts, ed., *Women, Health and Reproduction.* London: Routledge & Kegan Paul.

Bell, S. 1984. "Medical Perspectives on Gender and Science: The Case of DES." Paper presented at the Sixth Berkshire Conference, Smith College, Northampton, Mass.

Berliner, H. S. 1975. "A Larger Perspective on the Flexner Report." *International Journal of Health Services* 5, no. 4:573–92.

Betts, D. 1975. "Still Life With Fruit." In P. Rotter, ed., *Bitches and Sad Ladies.* New York: Dell. First printed 1973.

Bleier, R. 1984. *Science and Gender: A Critique of Biology and Its Theories on Women.* New York: Pergamon Press.

Bok, D. 1984. *The President's Report, 1982–83.* Cambridge, Mass.: Harvard University.

Bosk, C. 1979. *Forgive and Remember: Managing Medical Failure.* Chicago: University of Chicago Press.

Boston Women's Health Book Collective. 1985. *The New Our Bodies, Ourselves.* New York: Simon and Schuster.

Braverman, H. 1974. *Labor and Monopoly Capital: The Degradation of Labor in the Twentieth Century.* New York: Monthly Review Press.

Breen, D. 1975. *The Birth of a First Child: Towards an Understanding of Femininity.* London: Tavistock.

Brighton Women and Science Group. 1980. *Alice Through the Microscope: The Power of Science Over Women's Lives.* London: Virago.

Broad, W., and N. Wade. 1982. *Betrayers of the Truth: Fraud and Deceit in the Halls of Science.* New York: Simon and Schuster.

Brodsky, A. 1985. Presentation on midwifery. Suffolk University, Boston.

Bursztajn, H., R. I. Feinbloom, R. M. Hamm, and A. Brodsky. 1981. *Medical Choices, Medical Chances: How Patients, Families and Physicians Can Cope With Uncertainty.* New York: Seymour Lawrence/Delacorte.

Byrne, P. S., and B. E. Long. 1976. *Doctors Talking to Patients.* London: Her Majesty's Stationery Office.

Cacciari, C. 1984. "Problem Presentation Rituals in Gynecological Consultation." In V. D'Urso and P. Leonardi, eds., *Discourse Analysis and Natural Rhetorics.* Padua: Cleup Publishers.

Cartwright, A. 1967. *Patients and Their Doctors.* London: Routledge & Kegan Paul.

Charney, E., R. Bynum, G. Eldredge, et al. 1967. "How Well Do Patients Take Oral Penicillin? A Collaborative Study in Private Practice." *Pediatrics* 40:188–95.

Cheever, S. 1987. *Doctors and Women.* New York: Clarkson N. Potter.

Chomsky, N. 1968. *Language and Mind.* New York: Harcourt Brace Jovanovich.

Cobb, B. 1954. "Why Do People Detour to Quacks?" *Psychiatric Bulletin* 3:66–69.

Conrad, P., and R. Kern, eds. 1986. *The Sociology of Health and Illness: Critical Perspectives,* 2d ed. New York: St. Martin's Press.

Corea, G. 1977. *The Hidden Malpractice.* New York: Jove/Harcourt Brace Jovanovich.

Cousins, N. 1979. *Anatomy of an Illness.* New York: Norton.

Culpepper, E. 1978. "Exploring Menstrual Attitudes." In M. S. Hennifin, ed., *Women Look at Biology Looking at Women.* Cambridge, Mass.: Schenckman.

Curran, W. J. 1984. "Medical Intelligence, Law-Medicine Notes." *New England Journal of Medicine* 310:704–5.

D'Andrade, R. A. n.d. "A Tentative Cultural Classification of Speech Acts." Unpublished manuscript. Department of Anthropology, University of California, San Diego.

Descartes, R. 1960. *Discourse on Method* and *Meditations.* Translated with an introduction by L. J. LaFleur. New York: Liberal Arts Press.

DiMatteo, M. R., and D. D. DiNicola. 1981. "Sources of Assessment of Physician Performance: A Study of Comparative Reliability and Patterns of Intercorrelation." *Medical Care* 8:829–42.

Doerr, H. 1984. *Stones for Ibarra.* New York: Viking Press.

Doyal, L. 1983. "Women, Health and the Sexual Division of Labor: A Case Study of the Women's Health Movement in Britain." *International Journal of Health Services* 13, no. 3:373–87.

Doyal, L., with I. Pennell. 1979. *The Political Economy of Health*. Boston: South End Press.

Drossman, D. A. 1983. "The Physician and the Patient: Review of the Psychosocial Gastrointestinal Literature With an Integrated Approach to the Patient." In M. H. Sleisenger and J. S. Fordran, eds., *Gastrointestinal Disease Pathophysiology Diagnosis Management*. Philadelphia: W. B. Saunders.

Duff, R., and A. Hollingshead. 1968. *Sickness and Society*. New York: Harper & Row.

Ehrenreich, B., and J. Ehrenreich. 1971. *The American Health Empire: Power, Profits and Politics*. New York: Vintage.

Ehrenreich, B., and D. English. 1978. *For Her Own Good: 150 Years of the Experts' Advice to Women*. Garden City, N.Y.: Anchor Books.

Ehrenreich, J. 1978. *The Cultural Crisis of Modern Medicine*. New York: Monthly Review Press.

Emerson, J. 1970. "Behavior in Private Places: Sustaining Definitions of Reality in Gynecological Examinations." In H. P. Dreitzel, ed., *Recent Sociology*. No. 2. New York: Macmillan.

Engel, G. L. 1977. "The Need for a New Medical Model: A Challenge for Biomedicine." *Science* 196 (April 8): 129–36.

Epstein, S. S. 1981. "The Political and Economic Basis of Cancer." In P. Conrad and R. Kern, eds., *The Sociology of Health and Illness: Critical Perspectives*. New York: St. Martin's Press.

Fee, E. 1983. "Women's Nature and Scientific Objectivity." In M. Lowe and R. Hubbard, eds., *Women's Nature: Rationalizations of Inequality*. New York: Pergamon Press.

Fisher, S. 1986. *In the Patient's Best Interests: The Politics of Women's Health Care*. New Brunswick, N.J.: Rutgers University Press.

Fisher, S., and A. D. Todd. 1986. "Friendly Persuasion: The Negotiation of Decisions to Use Oral Contraceptives." In S. Fisher and A. Todd, eds., *Discourse and Institutional Authority: Medicine, Education, and Law*. Norwood, N.J.: Ablex.

———, eds. 1983. *The Social Organization of Doctor-Patient Communication*. Washington, D.C.: Center for Applied Linguistics/Harcourt Brace Jovanovich.

Frankel, R. 1983. "The Laying on of Hands: Aspects of the Organization of Gaze, Touch, and Talk in a Medical Encounter." In S. Fisher and A. D. Todd, eds., *The Social Organization of Doctor-Patient Communication*. Washington, D.C.: Center for Applied Linguistics/Harcourt Brace Jovanovich.

Freidson, E. 1970. *Professional Dominance*. Chicago: Aldine.

Funkenstein, D. H. 1978. *Medical Students, Medical Schools, and Society During Five Eras*, Cambridge, Mass.: Ballinger.

Gardner, K. 1981. "Well Woman Clinics: A Positive Approach to Women's Health." In H. Roberts, ed., *Women, Health and Reproduction*. London: Routledge & Kegan Paul.

Garfinkel, H. 1967. *Studies in Ethnomethodology*. Englewood Cliffs, N.J.: Prentice-Hall.

Gilligan, C. 1982. *In a Different Voice: Psychological Theory and Women's Development*. Cambridge, Mass.: Harvard University Press.

Goldsmith, J. C. 1981. *Can Hospitals Survive: The New Competitive Health Care Market*. Homewood, Ill.: Dow Jones–Irwin.

Gordon, J. S. 1984. "Holistic Health Centers in the United States." In J. W. Salmon, ed., *Alternative Medicines: Popular and Policy Perspectives*. New York: Tavistock.

Gordon, L. 1976. *Woman's Body, Woman's Right*. New York: Penguin Books.

Gorton, D. A. 1890. "Natural Psychology." In *Mental and Nervous Diseases*. In New York State Commission in Lunacy, *Miscellaneous Documents*, 37.

Gould, S. J. 1981. *The Mismeasure of Man*. New York: Norton.

Graham, H., and A. Oakley. 1981. "Competing Ideologies of Reproduction: Medical and Maternal Perspectives in Pregnancy." In H. Roberts, ed., *Women, Health and Reproduction*. London: Routledge & Kegan Paul.

Harding, S. 1986. *The Science Question in Feminism*. Ithaca, N.Y.: Cornell University Press.

Harraway, D. J. 1981. "In the Beginning Was the Word: The Genesis of Biological Theory." *Signs* 6, no. 3: 469–81.

Harrington, M. 1984. *The New American Poverty*. New York: Penguin Books.

Hauser, S. T. 1981. "Physician-Patient Relationships." In E. G. Mishler et al., *Social Contexts of Health, Illness, and Patient Care*. Cambridge: Cambridge University Press.

Hilfiker, D. 1984. "Sounding Board, Facing Our Mistakes." *New England Journal of Medicine* 310:118–22.

———. 1985. *Healing the Wounds*. New York: Pantheon.

Hingson, R., N. A. Scotch, J. Sorenson, and J. P. Swazey. 1981. *In Sickness and in Health: Social Dimensions of Medical Care*. St. Louis: Mosby.

Hubbard, R. 1983. "Social Effects of Some Contemporary Myths About Women." In M. Lowe and R. Hubbard, eds., *Woman's Nature: Rationalizations of Inequality*. New York: Pergamon Press.

Hulka, B., J. Cassel, L. Kupper, and J. Purdette. 1976. "Communication, Compliance and Concordance Between Physicians and Patients With Prescribed Medication." *American Journal of Public Health* 66: 847–53.

Hymes, D. 1972. "Models of the Interaction of Language and Social Life." In J. Gumperz and D. Hymes, eds., *Directions in Sociolinguistics: The Ethnography of Communication*. New York: Holt, Rinehart and Winston.

Ingelfinger, F. J. 1977. "Health: A Matter of Statistics or Feeling?" *New England Journal of Medicine* 296:448–49.

Jacobs, P. 1978. "Planned Parenthood Workers Likely to Shun the Pill." *Los Angeles Times*, Oct. 26.

Jaggar, A. M. 1983. *Feminist Politics and Human Nature*. Totowa, N.J.: Rowman and Allanheld.

Janis, I. L. 1958. *Psychological Stress: Psychoanalytic and Behavioral Studies of Surgical Patients*. New York: Wiley.

Jansen, M. A. 1987. "Women's Health Issues: An Emerging Priority for Health Psychology." In G. Stone et al., eds., *Health Psychology: A Discipline and a Profession*. Chicago: University of Chicago Press.

Jarnfelt, A. 1982. Paper presented at the World Congress of Gynecology and Obstetrics. Women and Health Roundtable report, session 10.

Johnson, J. E. 1966. "The Influence of Purposeful Nurse-Patient Interaction on the Patient's Postoperative Course." ANA Monograph Series No. 2: *Exploring Medical-Surgical Nursing Practice*. New York: American Nurses' Association.

———. 1975. "Stress Reduction through Sensation Information." In I. Sarason and C. Spielberger, eds., *Stress and Anxiety*. Vol. 2. New York: Wiley.

Johnson, J. E., and H. Leventhal. 1974. "Effects of Accurate Expectations and Behavioral Instructions on Reactions During a Noxious Medical Examination." *Journal of Personality and Social Psychology* 29: 710–18.

Keller, E. F. 1983. *A Feeling for the Organism*. San Francisco: Freeman.

———. 1983. "Gender and Science." In S. Harding and M. B. Hintikka, eds., *Discovering Reality: Feminist Perspectives on Epistemology, Metaphysics, Methodology, and Philosophy of Science*. Boston: D. Reidel.

———. 1985. *Reflections on Gender and Science*. New Haven: Yale University Press.

Kleinman, A. 1980. *Patients and Healers in the Context of Culture*. Berkeley and Los Angeles: University of California Press.

Knox, R. 1984. *The Boston Globe*, October 21.

Knox, R. 1984. *The Boston Globe*, November 29.

Knox, R., and M. Karagianis. 1984. *The Boston Globe*, October 21.

Kohlberg, L. 1981. *The Philosophy of Moral Development*. San Francisco: Harper & Row.

Korsch, B. M., E. Gozzi, and V. Francis. 1968. "Gaps in Doctor-Patient Communications." *Pediatrics* 42:846.

Korsch, B. M., and V. F. Negrete. 1972. "Doctor-Patient Communication." *Scientific American* 227:66–74.

Knorr-Cetina, K. D. 1981. *The Manufacture of Knowledge: An Essay on the Constructivist and Contextual Nature of Science*. New York: Pergamon Press.

Kuhns, W. 1971. *The Post-Industrial Prophets: Interpretations of Technology*. New York: Harper Colophon Books.

Labov, W., and D. Fanshel. 1977. *Therapeutic Discourse: Psychotherapy as Conversation*. New York: Academic Press.

Langer, E. J., I. L. Janis, and J. A. Wolfer. 1975. "Reduction of Psychological Stress in Surgical Patients." *Journal of Experimental Social Psychology* 11:155–65.

Langer, E. J., and J. Rodin. 1976. "The Effects of Choice and Enhanced Personal Responsibility for the Aged: A Field Experiment in an Institutional Setting." *Journal of Personality and Social Psychology* 34: 191–98.

Latour, B., and S. Woolgar. 1979. *Laboratory Life: Social Construction of Scientific Facts*. London: Sage.

Lavin, J. H. 1983. "Why 3 out of 5 Patients Switch." *Medical Economics*. May, pp. 11–17.

Lazarre, A., S. Eisenthal, and L. Wasserman. 1975. "The Customer Approach to Patienthood: Attending to Patients' Requests in a Walk-in Clinic." *Archives of General Psychiatry* 32:553–58.

Leavitt, J. W. 1984. *Women and Health in America*. Madison: University of Wisconsin Press.

Lennane, J. K., and J. R. Lennane. 1973. "Alleged Psychogenic Disorders in

Women—A Possible Manifestation of Sexual Prejudice." *New England Journal of Medicine* 288:289–92.

Levidow, L., and B. Young, eds. 1981. *Science, Technology, and the Labour Process.* London: Blockrose Press.

Levy, J. M., and R. K. McGee. 1975. "Childbirth as Crises: A Test of Janis' Theory of Communication and Stress Resolution." *Journal of Personality and Social Psychology* 31:171–79.

Luker, K. 1975. *Taking Chances.* Berkeley and Los Angeles: University of California Press.

———. 1984. *Abortion and the Politics of Motherhood.* Berkeley and Los Angeles: University of California Press.

MacCormack, C. P. 1980. "Nature, Culture and Gender: A Critique." In C. P. MacCormack and M. Strathern, eds., *Nature, Culture and Gender.* Cambridge: Cambridge University Press.

Marchasin, S. M. 1984. *Los Angeles Times,* August 1.

Martin, E. 1987. *The Woman in the Body: A Cultural Analysis of Reproduction.* Boston: Beacon Press.

Matchen, L. 1984. *The Boston Globe,* September 26.

McKeown, T. 1976. *The Role of Medicine: Dream, Mirage, or Nemesis?* London: Nullfield Provincial Hospitals Trust.

McKinlay, J. B. 1975. "Who Is Really Ignorant?" *Journal of Health and Social Behavior* 16:3–11.

———. 1981. "From 'Promising Report' to 'Standard Procedure': Seven Stages in the Career of a Medical Innovation." *Milbank Memorial Fund Quarterly/Health and Society* 59, no. 3:233–70.

Mechanic, D. 1968. *Medical Sociology.* New York: Free Press. 2d ed. 1978.

Mehan, H. 1979. *Learning Lessons.* Cambridge, Mass.: Harvard University Press.

Mehl, L. E. 1977. "Research in Childbirth Alternatives: What Can It Tell Us About Hospital Practice?" In L. Stewart and D. Stewart, eds., *21st Century Obstetrics Now!* Chapel Hill: NAPSAC.

Merchant, C. 1980. *The Death of Nature: Women, Ecology and the Scientific Revolution.* San Francisco: Harper & Row.

Merton, R. K. 1973. *The Sociology of Science.* Chicago: University of Chicago Press.

Messing, K. 1983. "The Scientific Mystique: Can a White Lab Coat Guarantee Purity in the Search for Knowledge About the Nature of Women?" In M. Lowe and R. Hubbard, eds., *Woman's Nature: Rationalizations of Inequality.* New York: Pergamon Press.

Miller, J. 1976. *Toward a New Psychology of Women.* Boston: Beacon Press.

Mishler, E. G. 1981. "Viewpoint: Critical Perspectives of the Biomedical Model." In E. G. Mishler et al., *Social Contexts of Health, Illness, and Patient Care.* Cambridge: Cambridge University Press.

———. 1984. *The Discourse of Medicine.* Norwood, N.J.: Ablex.

Mishler, E. G., L. R. AmaraSingham, S. T. Hauser, R. Liem, S. D. Osherson, and N. E. Waxler. 1981. *Social Contexts of Health, Illness, and Patient Care.* Cambridge: Cambridge University Press.

Mumford, E., H. J. Schlesinger, and G. V. Glass. 1982. "The Effect of Psychological Intervention on Recovery from Surgery and Heart Attacks: An Analysis of the Literature." *American Journal of Public Health* 72:141–51.

Navarro, V. 1976. *Medicine Under Capitalism*. New York: Prodist.
———. 1986. *Crisis, Health and Medicine: A Social Critique*. New York: Tavistock.
O'Brien, M. 1981. *The Politics of Reproduction*. London: Routledge & Kegan Paul.
Okin, S. M. 1979. *Women in Western Political Thought*. Princeton: Princeton University Press.
Osherson, S., and L. AmaraSingham. 1981. "The Machine Metaphor in Medicine." In E. G. Mishler et al., *Social Contexts of Health, Illness, and Patient Care*. Cambridge: Cambridge University Press.
Paget, M. A. 1983. "On the Work of Talk: Studies in Misunderstandings." In S. Fisher and A. D. Todd, eds., *The Social Organization of Doctor-Patient Communication*. Washington, D.C.: Center for Applied Linguistics/Harcourt Brace Jovanovich.
Parachini, A. 1984. *Los Angeles Times*, July 27.
Parsons, T. 1951. *The Social System*. New York: Free Press.
Petchesky, R. P. 1985. "Abortion in the 1980's: Feminist Morality and Women's Health." In E. Lewin and V. Oleson, eds., *Women, Health and Healing: Toward a New Perspective*. New York: Tavistock.
Powles, J. 1973. "On the Limitations of Modern Medicine." *Science, Medicine and Man* 1:1–30.
Prather, J., and L. Fidell. 1975. "Sex Differences in the Content and Style of Medical Advertisements." *Social Science and Medicine* 9 (Jan.): 23–26.
Preston, T. 1981. *The Clay Pedestal*. Seattle: Madrona Publishers.
Ray, I. 1866. "The Insanity of Woman Produced by Desertion or Seduction." *American Journal of Insanity* 23:272.
Reiser, S. J. 1978. *Medicine and the Reign of Technology*. Cambridge: Cambridge University Press.
Rhys, J. 1960. "Outside the Machine." In J. Rhys, *Tigers Are Better Looking*. New York: Popular Library.
Rich, A. 1976. *Of Woman Born: Motherhood as Experience and Institution*. New York: Norton.
Riessman, C. K. 1983. "Women and Medicalization: A New Perspective." *Social Policy* 14 (Summer): 3–18.
Risen, R. 1984. *Los Angeles Times*, August 16.
Rodin, J. 1982. "Patient-Practitioner Relationships: A Process of Social Influence." In A. W. Johnson et al., eds., *Contemporary Health Services: Social Science Perspectives*. Boston: Auburn House.
Rose, H., and S. Rose. 1969. *Science and Society*. London: Penguin Press.
Rothman, B. K. 1982. *In Labor: Women and Power in the Birthplace*. New York: Norton.
Rusek, S. 1978. *The Women's Health Movement*. New York: Praeger.
Sacks, H., E. Schegloff, and G. Jefferson, 1974. "A Simplest Systematics for the Analysis of Turn Taking in Conversation." *Language* 50:7–55.
Scheff, T. 1968. "Negotiating Reality: Notes on Power in the Assessment of Responsibility." *Social Problems* 16:3–17.
Schiefelbein, S. 1980. "The Female Patient: Heeded? Hustled? Healed?" *Saturday Review*, March 29.
Scull, A. T., and D. Favreau. 1986. "'A Chance to Cut Is a Chance to Cure': Sexual Surgery for Psychosis in Three Nineteenth Century Societies."

In S. Spitzer and A. T. Scull, eds., *Research in Law, Deviance and Social Control*, 8:3–39. Greenwich, Conn.: JAI Press.

Scully, D. 1980. *Men Who Control Women's Health: The Miseducation of Obstetrician-Gynecologists*. Boston: Houghton Mifflin.

Scully, D., and P. Bart. 1973. "A Funny Thing Happened on the Way to the Orifice: Women in Gynecology Textbooks." *American Journal of Sociology* 78 (Jan.):1045–50.

Seaman, B. 1969. *The Doctors' Case Against the Pill.* 2d ed., 1980. New York: Avon.

Searle, J. R. 1969. *Speech Acts: An Essay in the Philosophy of Language.* Cambridge: Cambridge University Press.

Segal, D. 1984. "Playing Doctor, Seriously: Graduation Follies at an American Medical School." *International Journal of Health Services* 14, no. 3: 379–97.

Shaw, G. B. 1909. *The Doctor's Dilemma.* In *Plays*, vol. 12. New York: William H. Wise.

Sherer, J. 1979. "Critical Theory, Hermeneutics, and the Analysis of Discourse." Unpublished paper, Sociology Department, University of California, San Diego.

Shryock, R. 1962. *Medicine and Society in America, 1660–1860.* Ithaca, N.Y.: Cornell University Press.

Shuy, R. 1974. "Problems of Communication in the Cross-Cultural Medical Interview." *Working Papers: Sociolinguistics.* No. 19. Washington, D.C.

———. 1983. "Three Types of Interference to an Effective Exchange of Information in the Medical Interview." In S. Fisher and A. D. Todd, eds., *The Social Organization of Doctor-Patient Communication.* Washington, D.C.: Center for Applied Linguistics/Harcourt Brace Jovanovich.

Sidel, V. W., and R. Sidel, eds., 1984. *Reforming Medicine: Lessons of the Last Quarter Century.* New York: Pantheon Books.

Siegler, M., and H. Osmond. 1974. *Models of Madness, Models of Medicine.* New York: Harper Colophon Books.

Silverman, D. 1984. "Going Private: Ceremonial Forms in a Private Oncology Clinic." *Sociology* 18 (May):191–204.

Silverman, D., and B. Torode. 1980. *The Material World.* London: Routledge & Kegan Paul.

Sloan, D., S. Shapiro, D. Kaufman, L. Rosenberg, O. Miettinen, and P. Stolley. 1981. "Risk of Myocardial Infarction in Relation to Current and Discontinued Use of Oral Contraceptives." *New England Journal of Medicine* 305:420–24.

Smith, D. 1974. "Women's Perspective as a Radical Critique of Sociology." *Sociological Inquiry* 4:7–13.

Smith-Rosenberg, C., and C. Rosenberg. 1984. "The Female Animal: Medical and Biological Views of Women and Her Role in Nineteenth-Century America." In J. W. Leavitt, ed., *Women and Health in America.* Madison: University of Wisconsin Press.

Starr, P. 1982. *The Social Transformation of American Medicine.* New York: Basic Books.

Stevens, R. 1971. *American Medicine and the Public Interest.* New Haven: Yale University Press.

Stiles, W. B., et al. 1979. "Interaction Exchange Structure and Patient Satisfaction With Medical Interviews," *Medical Care* 17:667–69.

Stone, G. C. 1979. "Patient Compliance and the Role of the Expert." *Journal of Social Issues* 35:34–59.

Storer, H. R. 1871. *The Causation, Course and Treatment of Reflex Insanity in Women.* Boston: Lee and Shephard.

Streeck, J. 1980. "Speech Acts in Interaction: A Critique of Searle." *Discourse Processes* 3:133–54.

Strong, P. M. 1979. *The Ceremonial Order of the Clinic: Parents, Doctors and Medical Bureaucracies.* London: Routledge & Kegan Paul.

Symonds, A. 1983. "Emotional Conflicts of the Career Woman: Women in Medicine." *American Journal of Psychoanalysis* 43 (1):21–37.

Taylor, R. 1984. "Alternative Medicine and the Medical Encounter in Britain and the United States." In J. W. Solomon, ed., *Alternative Medicines: Popular and Policy Perspectives.* New York: Tavistock.

Todd, A. D. 1983. "Women's Bodies as Diseased and Deviant: Historical and Contemporary Issues." In S. Spitzer, ed., *Research in Law, Deviance and Social Control,* 5. Greenwich, Conn.: JAI Press.

———. 1984. "The Prescription of Contraception: Negotiations Between Doctors and Patients." *Discourse Processes* 7:171–200.

Treichler, P., R. M. Frankel, C. Kramarae, K. Zoppi, and H. B. Beckman. 1984. "Problems and *Problems:* Power Relations in a Medical Encounter." In C. Kramarae, M. Shulz, and W. M. O'Barr, eds., *Language and Power.* London: Sage.

Treichler, P., and C. Kramarae. 1984. "Medicine, Language and Women: Whose Body?" *Women and Language News* 7 (Spring):1–2.

Vaccarino, J. M. 1977. "Malpractice: The Problem in Perspective." *Journal of the American Medical Association* 238:861–63.

Vernon, D. T. A., and D. A. Bigelow. 1974. "Effect of Information About a Potentially Stressful Situation on Responses to Stress Impact." *Journal of Personality and Social Psychology* 29:50–59.

Waitzkin, H. B. 1983. *The Second Sickness: Contradictions of Capitalist Health Care.* New York: Free Press.

———. 1984. "Doctor-Patient Communication: Clinical Implications of Social Scientific Research." *Journal of the American Medical Association* 252:2441–46.

Waitzkin, H. B., and J. D. Stoeckle. 1972. "The Communication of Information About Illness." *Advanced Psychosomatic Medicine* 8:180.

Waitzkin, H. B., and B. Waterman. 1974. *The Exploitation of Illness in Capitalist Society.* Indianapolis: Bobbs-Merrill.

Wallen, J., H. Waitzkin, and J. D. Stoeckle. 1979. "Physician Stereotypes About Female Health and Illness: A Study of Patient's Sex and the Informative Process During Medical Interviews." *Women and Health* 4:135–46.

Weideger, P. 1975. *Menstruation and Menopause.* New York: Dell.

Wertz, R., and D. Wertz. 1977. *Lying-In: A History of Childbirth in America.* New York: Free Press.

Wertz, D. C., J. R. Sorenson, and T. C. Heeren. 1984. "Communication in Professional-Lay Encounters: How Often Do Both Parties Know What the Other Wants to Discuss?" Paper presented at the American Sociological Association, San Antonio.

West, C. 1984. *Routine Complications*. Bloomington: Indiana University Press.

Wolcott, I. 1979. "Women and Psychoactive Drug Use." *Women and Health* 4:199–202.

Wolfer, J. A., and M. A. Vistainer. 1975. "Pediatric Surgical Patients of Psychologic Preparation and Stress-Point Nursing Care." *Nursing Research* 24:244–55.

Wright, W. 1984. *The Social Logic of Health*. New Brunswick, N.J.: Rutgers University Press.

Wright, W. "Wild Knowledge: Natural Science and Social Theory in a Fragile Environment." Manuscript in progress. Memorial University of Newfoundland.

Zilsel, E. 1974. "The Sociological Roots of Science." In W. H. Truitt and T. W. G. Solomans, eds., *Science, Technology and Freedom*. Boston: Houghton Mifflin.

Zola, I. K. 1972. "Studying the Decisions to See a Doctor." In Z. S. Lipowski, ed., *Psychological Aspects of Physical Illness*, Vol. 8: *Advances in Psychosomatic Medicine*. Basel, Switzerland: S. Karger.

———. 1980. "Structural Constraints in the Doctor-Patient Relationship: The Case of Non-Compliance." In L. Eisenberg and A. Kleinman, eds., *The Relevance of Social Science and Medicine*. Boston: D. Reidel.

Index